THE
CORONA PROTOCOL
—PRESCRIBER'S GUIDE—

PAUL D. CORONA, M.D.

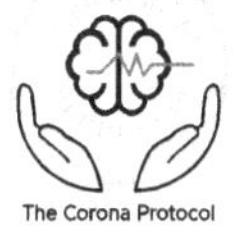

The Corona Protocol Prescriber's Guide
by Paul D. Corona, M.D.

Hardcover: 979-8-9998715-6-5
Paperback: 979-8-9998715-5-8
eBook: 979-8-9998715-7-2
LCCN: 2025923132
Published by The Corona Protocol,
    30011 Ivy Glenn Dr., Suite 101, Laguna Niguel, CA 92677

    www.drpaulcoronamd.com

All rights reserved. No part of this publication may be reproduced in any form, or by any means, electronic or mechanical, including photocopying, recording, or any information browsing, storage, or retrieval system, without permission in writing from the author.

Copyright © 2026 by Paul D. Corona, M.D.

Edited by Lisa Burnett
Cover Design: Jamie Simon
Author Photograph: Jackie Tran
Interior Design: Karen Corriente

First Printing Edition, 2026

Library of Congress Cataloguing-in-Publication
Corona, M.D., Paul D.
    The Corona Protocol Prescriber's Guide
    Paul D. Corona, M.D. p.288

Although this publication is designed to provide accurate information in regard to the subject matter covered, the publisher and the author assume no responsibility for errors, inaccuracies, omissions, or any other inconsistencies herein. This publication is meant as a source of valuable information for the reader, however it is not meant as a replacement for direct expert assistance. If such level of assistance is required, the services of a competent professional should be sought.

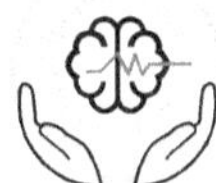

Acknowledgments

I want to thank my amazing assistant Leslie Perez, who goes above and beyond and is such a pleasure to work with every day in the office.

I want to acknowledge Lisa Burnett, who has not only edited these two books but also re-edited my first three books to be released as a second edition. I can't believe that she has never done professional book editing before, yet she has a gift for it. She is also my videographer for *The Dr. Paul Show* on Roku, Amazon Fire and YouTube. It has been a pleasure working with her on these projects.

Thank you to Karen Corriente for all her hard work doing the typesetting and layout not only for these two books but also for the second edition of my first three books *Healing the Mind and Body: The Trilogy.*

Thank you to Jaime Simon for the cover design of these two books as well as the second edition of my first three books.

Thank you to my patients who have taught me so much and have become friends. There is nothing I enjoy more than healing the minds and bodies of those that have entrusted me with their care.

Special thanks to my pastor, mentor and friend Chuck Smith Jr. who has helped me since the beginning of my writing journey 23 years ago. He has given me excellent advice and editing for most of my books.

Lastly I want to thank my father Arthur Corona, who has not only been incredibly supportive over the years but also has been a role model my whole life. Thank you to my wife Denise, my son Logan and my daughter Baylee. I also want to mention by best buddy and soul cat Seymour and our dog JG. I love you all very much.

TABLE OF CONTENTS

— CHAPTER ONE —

— CHAPTER TWO —

— CHAPTER THREE —

— CHAPTER FOUR —

— CHAPTER FIVE —

— CHAPTER SIX —

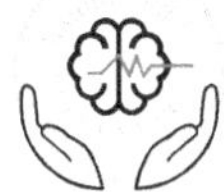

Introduction

I have written this brief guide to complement my first three books of the *Healing the Mind and Body* trilogy series, as well as the other two in *The Corona Protocol* book series. This is especially the case regarding my third book, which is mainly meant for healthcare providers who are clinicians and are able to prescribe psychotropic medications. This not only includes primary care physicians such as family practitioners, internists, and pediatricians, but also PAs (physician assistants), NPs (nurse practitioners), and, in rare cases, psychologists and pharmacists. This book is meant to be a clinical guide to help providers make rational treatment decisions based on the evidence at hand. Chapters 2 and 3 of my third book regarding psychotropic medications are very long and detailed, so it is meant to be a resource guide to be used by prescribers and is also meant to be a resource for psychologists, social workers, nurses, pharmacists, physical therapists, or any other profession that contributes to the care of these patients.

The book is also written for the layperson who is interested in more detailed information about my take on how best to treat issues regarding mental and physical health in order to improve our patients' lives. It also allows the layperson to get an inside look at how doctors think and make the decisions we do. The Internet can be a very confusing source of information about this topic as well as other medical issues. Besides the Internet, family and friends, pharmacists, and other sources of opinion regarding mental health concerns, which is way beyond their expertise. This usually causes more confusion and misinformation rather than revealing the real truth about mind-body disorders.

The purpose of this guide is to simplify and streamline the decision-making process regarding psychotropic-related treatment decisions in a rational algorithmic way. My hope is to be able to integrate the art of clinical practice with the science of psychopharmacology, which, when done properly, leads to the rational pharmaceutical approach to treatment that I advocate in my books. I sincerely believe that the field of mind-body medicine is the most cutting-edge and exciting field in medicine today. It is also the area of medicine that has the potential to make the biggest positive difference in the lives of the vast majority of our patients.

I started my writing journey about 2002 and released my first book at the end of 2007, then my second and third books between 2008 and 2014, when I released my 3-book series *Healing the Mind and Body: The Trilogy*. I then took a much-needed break from writing and switched to my other favorite pastime of reading, usually fantasy novels. After about a year or so in 2015, I got the itch and decided that I needed to write another book or two.

I had been thinking about this over the previous year before I decided to write again. I realized that I had learned so much, and it was apparent to me that what I had discovered was not common knowledge. I realized that I had learned new ways to diagnose and treat these conditions in ways that were not being done. I was frustrated because I had discovered that there were so many people that were suffering and not getting the help that they needed. I knew I needed to teach what I had learned with doctors and other providers, especially primary care providers such as myself, as well as psychiatrists that have an open mind to learning a new way of doing things that is different than what they learned in training and by reading their textbooks and journals. The first one is *The Corona Protocol: Three Secrets to Success*, and the second one is *The Corona Protocol: Prescriber's Guide*, the one that you are currently reading.

I then took a much-needed break again from writing and then started reading again, and then about a year later in 2020, I decided to write another book. I had been thinking about it over the previous year and really wanted to write something that was different. Since I have been a fiction fan my whole life, I wanted to write a book about storytelling regarding people who suffer with different types of mental illness. In 2024 I released *The Corona Protocol: A Scientifically Proven Medical Solution to STOP Addiction, Bullying, Homelessness, School Shootings, and Suicide, 30 years in the making*. This book was fun to write, even though writing a book is a lot of hard work, since I tell 30 original short stories about people that suffer with different types of mental and physical illnesses. The book is about half fiction and half nonfiction. I also tell my story and the last two sections of the book, which included my journey of discovery and how I learned what I learned each step of the way. I also share difficult times that I have gone through and how I was able to persevere.

After a short break I took out of storage the two previous teaching manuals that I had written and started editing them in order to release them in 2025. Also, between 2024 and

2025, I re-edited my first three books, *Healing the Mind and Body: The Trilogy,* in order to release them in 2025. The first two books of the trilogy are more for patients but also for doctors, while the third book of this series is more for doctors but also for patients. There have been new medications that have come out since these books were first released. I have added these medications along with details on how I prescribe them in the "Medications" chapter of the book. The re-editing was all accomplished by the middle of 2025. This has been a huge relief for me after writing six books over 23 years, since they have finished what I started. I have no further plans to write another book, except for a future fantasy series, but that will not be any time too soon.

In this book I will not be discussing dosing or titration strategies, which are available in my third book, as well as the first two, which cover the basic concepts and theories regarding psychotropic medications. In the third book, though, I more comprehensively discuss how to take a complete history in chapter 1, and I provide detailed instructions regarding treatment issues in chapter 4, such as augmentation strategies, how long to take medications, and many other practical issues for the prescriber. In chapter 5 I review in detail several case studies to show how it all comes together regarding the care of different individuals.

The exciting aspect of this field of medicine is that newer and even better breakthroughs will continue. In this book, I will focus more on the practical aspects of clinical treatment in this area of medicine. I will attempt to simplify the concepts in this book on purpose so that it is practical and easy to follow and understand. My goal is to make this book as short as I can while still attempting to be as complete as I need it to be. I want to stress that I'm sharing the way that I assess and treat patients at this time, but this is a burgeoning and cutting-edge field of medicine, so we are constantly learning newer and better ways of helping patients achieve their goals.

As newer and even better medications come out, I attempt to improve my techniques while searching for better results with the least, or even no, side effects. However, it's important to stress that all of the medications that are currently available are more than adequate to get the vast majority of patients completely better. It's still nice, though, when new options become available to be explored. Trigger warning: There are many opinions and recommendations in this book as well as my previous and current ones that may conflict and disagree with other books available on this topic. Much of my protocol, if not most, is based on "off-label" prescribing, which is simply the most cutting-edge method in this field of medicine.

These are my personal opinions based on a lot of practical experience from practicing over the last more than three decades. (That is why it is called a medical practice, since we keep practicing until we get it right.) I will be as honest as I can, even if my views are not politically correct and disagree with other opinions, including in particular the FDA, the CDC, or whichever governmental body. Newer and exciting breakthroughs will continue to occur, such as new technologies, diagnostic strategies, and even better medications, as well as more current non-pharmacological therapies. There is nothing more exciting about being a doctor than witnessing patients experiencing dramatic results and improvements in their quality of life. That's why we do what we do.

One of my favorite authors is Malcolm Gladwell. In two of his books, he writes about a couple of concepts that really affected me personally and professionally. In *Outliers* he discusses why he claims that "10,000 is the magic number of greatness." By his research he found out that it takes 10,000 hours of practice in order to gain mastery of a field. Practicing early and often, combined with knowledge and expertise, leads to the most desired results. That's why we call it a clinical practice, since we are simply practicing in order to learn how to do things in the best way. What's exciting about this field of medicine is that even after well over 60,000 hours of practicing (10,000 hours is about five years of clinical practice), there is still so much left for me to learn. Doctors and other providers never stop learning, which is why this profession is so challenging, satisfying, and fun.

In his second book, *Blink*, one of my favorites, Malcolm discusses the fascinating subject of *thin-slicing,* which refers to the ability of the unconscious to find patterns in situations and behaviors based on very narrow slices and windows of experience. This leads to more fine-tuned instincts when we explore the power of the unconscious mind, which then more efficiently leads to the results that we are ultimately seeking. Einstein said, "The only real valuable thing is intuition." Intuition is a sense of knowing something without going through all the stages, steps, and proofs to reach a conclusion. An experienced physician may take 5 to 10 minutes to reach a diagnosis and treatment strategy, while the doctor in training or early in practice may take hours or even days to reach the same conclusions, if at all. The experienced brain is able to selectively access its complete store of knowledge along with multiple associations with familiar situations from the past, as well as other pertinent pieces of information gained from experience, creativity, and reason. *Thin-slicing* is educated intuition in action. Malcolm refers to this as "thinking without thinking."

In order to use this method, I have every new patient fill out my New Patient form on my website before he or she sees me in the office. In this form I ask detailed questions regarding every area of health that I want to address. Within a few minutes of reading this information, I am able to learn a great deal about that patient, such as detailed current and past symptomatology, a complete family history, the details regarding previous medications tried and failed, the course of the illness, as well as other information that is important in order to get a complete assessment of that patient. Then, when I spend that first hour or so with the patient, I am able to make quick and accurate decisions by *thin-slicing* and thus picking out the most important pieces of information, which, when taken together, helps to guide me to be able to make the best treatment decisions by the rational trial-and-error treatment approach.

CHAPTER ONE

The Neurochemical Imbalances

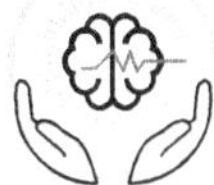

The Neurochemical Imbalances

In this book I will present different types of patients that we clinicians see quite commonly, and then I will discuss how I go about evaluating them and then how I go about deciding how to start treatment and how I decide what to do on the second visit, the third visit, and beyond. Our goal is to get each patient completely well, defined as achieving and maintaining *full remission* for each individual. I will be listing "formal" definitions of many mind-body disorders from the DSM-IV and DSM-5. I'm not doing this just to bore you, but rather to highlight the similarities and differences between the formally established mood disorders. As you will see, there is a lot of overlap of symptoms between these defined disorders, so you will see that it can be difficult to fit an individual patient with an individual's story and needs into a nice neat tidy box of a diagnosis. It's not very common in clinical practice to see "pure" diagnoses that do not overlap with other diagnoses.

Most patients have a combination of different symptoms and problems that do not always fit neatly into established categories and definitions. This is why it is important to look at the bigger picture when it comes to assessing each patient. Each person and presentation is unique, with no two exactly the same, so the challenge for clinicians is to evaluate and treat each patient with an individualized assessment and treatment plan by listening intently, practicing, and then trying our best to get it right.

For example, let's say you see a patient with major depressive disorder (MDD), social anxiety disorder (SAD), intermittent panic attacks, insomnia (both difficulty falling asleep and staying asleep), headaches, and persistent fatigue. How do we decide how to go about treating someone with this presentation? What do we do first? What do we do second and third? Do we treat one issue at a time or approach them all together? The typical psychiatric approach is to first focus on the Axis 1 diagnosis and to pick an FDA-approved medication that is indicated for that diagnosis. (As you probably know by now, I do not care what the FDA or any governmental body thinks about how to make clinical decisions in this field of medicine.) Which primary Axis 1 diagnosis would you choose first? Does the way that you approach treating that depend on the other diagnoses the patient has?

My best advice is to look at the whole person and all the diagnoses together, as well as getting a full and complete history, with a complete review of systems, before deciding what to do first, second, and beyond. I also decide what treatment I think will work best, not just what is government-approved to be used for a certain indication. I would prescribe a medication based on how many of these diagnoses can be treated together in the most complete way. Based on the response to the first medication, I can then assess whether it was the right choice or not and then see what is left over in order to decide which augmentation strategy to choose.

Let's discuss some other examples of individuality. How about a patient who presents with generalized anxiety disorder (GAD), dysthymia (depression-lite), ADHD, irritable bowel syndrome (IBS), obsessive-compulsive disorder (OCD), hypochondriasis, and narcissistic personality disorder? How about a patient with bipolar II disorder, PTSD, fibromyalgia, chronic fatigue syndrome (CFS), and borderline personality disorder (BPD)? How about someone with cyclothymic disorder (hypomania with hypodepression), recurring migraine and tension headaches, premenstrual dysphoric disorder (PMDD), and anxiety attacks? How about a tough one like a patient with Bipolar I Disorder, severe ADHD, and a distant history of methamphetamine abuse?

These are the types of presentations that are commonly seen by us treating providers on a daily basis. How do we tackle treating a patient who has so many coexisting disorders, personality types, and psychological stressors all at the same time? As I said, the approach I advocate is to look at the big picture by taking in all of the factors together all at the same time. I advocate the history-based and symptom-based approach by gathering as much information as possible, and then we can make our best guesses as to which neurochemical or combination of neurochemicals are imbalanced and in need of being properly fine-tuned. In most cases, especially more complicated cases, there are more than one of the neurochemicals in need of being balanced properly. Usually there are at least two, but more likely three, four, or more that need attending to. The body and mind don't really care how many medications it takes. It just wants to feel better, and it's well worth the wait once the results are realized.

My habit that I have found very useful is that I have every new patient call me a week after the visit to report to me the results of the intervention. I can usually tell within the first week whether I chose the right medication or not. If not then, I can change it prior to the visit. I typically titrate the medication as quickly and safely as possible in order to get to the best dosage before I move on. Being in touch with patients after the first visit and between other visits is an excellent customer service secret. It shows patients that I care, which I most certainly do. I also return every phone call and every email the same day. These are great tips for retaining clients who are not used to such personalized care.

After the first intervention I can then assess whether I was right or not based on the response. I then either decide to change it to something potentially better or to continue it and augment it with another. I make these decisions during and in-between visits (by getting updates over the phone before the following visit) as I hear more detailed information in order to best help my patients. I then continue this approach each visit until full remission is achieved and maintained over time.

We need to acknowledge that the method we have of picking which psychotropic agent to use is by trial-and-error, but it is *rational* trial-and-error. We make our best guesstimates based on the most detailed and complete information that we have available to us. I have found that it is important to be wrong on occasion before we learn to do what is right. We learn from our mistakes. This should not be surprising, though, since science of any type is also based on trial and error. This is the case in every specialty regarding every aspect of clinical medicine, as well as life itself for that matter.

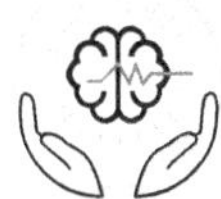

The Critical Importance of the First Step

It is important to get the first medication right before considering augmenting. If the results are okay but not great, then I would switch to something potentially better in order to see if it is. It may take more than one or two tries before the correct initial or augmenting medication is chosen, but it is worth the time and effort in order to get it right before we move on. That's the error part of trial-and-error, and it is a necessary part on the road to learning the truth.

If my choice is wrong, then I evaluate the details of any positive results as well as negative results and side effects. This information then gives me clues in order to reconsider the diagnosis and approach treatment in a different way. We need to keep our minds open to reconsider the diagnosis and treatment approach as we learn more by working closely with our patients and keeping the lines of communication open, especially by being good listeners, which is the most important aspect in communication. The more we hear from patients and get to know them, the better we understand them, and the better we are then able to help them to achieve their goals.

As I alluded to earlier, it is rare that one medication alone is enough to get the patient completely well by achieving the ultimate goal of full remission for each person. Some patients who only have an imbalance of serotonin do perfectly well with an SSRI and don't need anything else, though that is not typical for most. Serotonin is often involved at some level, though more often than not it is not imbalanced on its own. There are more often than not 2-4 neurochemical imbalances at one time, requiring 2-3 medications on average in order to create the proper balance. It really doesn't matter how many medications or non-pharmacological interventions it takes in order to attend to the complete needs of the individual. The body and mind don't really care what it takes in order to feel better, since it's worth it once the results are realized.

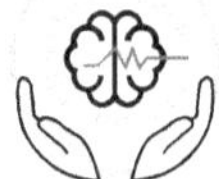

The Fantastic Four

Let's briefly review the four neurochemicals that I refer to as "The Fantastic Four." They are serotonin, norepinephrine, dopamine, and GABA/glutamate. Serotonin is more often than not involved with patients who have depression or anxiety disorders. However, it's usually not imbalanced on its own, and in some it may not be a factor at all. If serotonin is imbalanced, then we also need to consider whether norepinephrine is as well. The basic choice to make is between an SSRI and an SNRI when treating unipolar depression, anxiety disorders, somatic symptoms, and others. I have found that an SNRI is more often than not a better choice than an SSRI, while the most common practice by most providers is to use an SSRI first-line, which is what most of the literature recommends. I have rather found, though, that an SSRI may be good, but an SNRI is usually better. It's just playing the odds, which makes more sense.

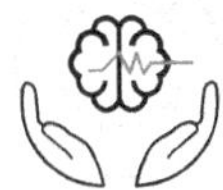

Serotonin

It's difficult to simplify how to recognize which neurochemical or neurochemicals are imbalanced based on history and examination. When I list symptoms related to an imbalance of whichever neurochemical, it's difficult to generalize since there are such a variety of potential presentations, but I will try. The key symptoms related to an imbalance of serotonin that I consider are symptoms of depression, symptoms of anxiety, worry, rumination, obsessive thinking, PMDD/PMS, insomnia (especially early-morning awakening and difficulty getting back to sleep), postpartum depression, OCD, and eating disorders, as well as others. Side effects of SSRIs include fatigue, apathy, sexual side effects, weight gain, nausea, activation, and others. The SSRIs currently available are Prozac (fluoxetine), Zoloft (sertraline), Paxil (paroxetine), Celexa (citalopram), Luvox (fluvoxamine), and Lexapro (escitalopram), along with the "super" SSRIs Viibryd (vilazodone) and Trintellix (vortioxetine).

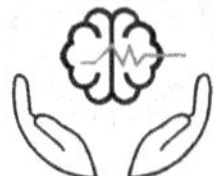

Norepinephrine

The key symptoms related to an imbalance of norepinephrine are symptoms of depression, symptoms of anxiety, somatic symptoms such as pain and other physical complaints, insomnia (especially difficulty shutting down and getting to sleep), fatigue, and difficulty with focus and concentration, as well as others. There is often an overlap between these two neurochemicals, which is why an SNRI more often than not provides more complete results than SSRIs. Side effects related to SNRIs include dry mouth, nausea, constipation, urinary retention, activation, fatigue, insomnia, sexual side effects (though less than SSRIs), and others. The reality, though, is that usually the side effects are mild or nonexistent. The SNRIs currently available are Effexor XR (venlafaxine ER), Cymbalta (duloxetine), Pristiq ER (desvenlafaxine succinate ER), and Fetzima (levomilnacipran). Others that affect these two neurochemicals are Remeron (mirtazapine), Serzone (nefazodone), and the tricyclic antidepressants.

Strattera (atomoxetine) was the first NRI (norepinephrine reuptake inhibitor), which not only balances norepinephrine but also dopamine slightly. This product has been generic for many years. The newest and second NRI, released the year that this book was released, is Qelbree (viloxazine). We cannot only slightly balance dopamine like Strattera (atomoxetine) does but also slightly balance serotonin. These non-stimulants not only help with ADD/ADHD but also can improve anxiety, somatic symptoms, and depressive symptoms. Wellbutrin is an NDRI, which is a dual-action agent in a sense, though it focuses more on dopamine than it does on norepinephrine.

It may be helpful to try both classes separately before deciding on which class, by letting the body decide which is best. If an SSRI is working okay but gives incomplete results that are not improved adequately even with increasing the dose, then it is time to move on and try something potentially better. If an SSRI works well initially but then the efficacy decreases over time even with adequate titration, I refer to this as the "Serotonin Poop-Out Syndrome." I have seen this very frequently over the years, and the problem is that doctors often get stuck on serotonin and try one SSRI after another. This bothers me to no end. I have found that it is better to keep an open mind and switch to a different class sooner rather than later.

If an SNRI provides excellent results, then there is probably no need to try an SSRI. However, if an SNRI does not clearly give better results than an SSRI in a short period of time, or if the noradrenergic side effects are too prominent, then I would consider switching back to an SSRI if it was chosen first, or if an SNRI was chosen before an SSRI. It's worth it to try different medications, whether in a different class or different ones in the same class, in order to make sure the best choice is made. The key is finding the best medication with the least or no side effects. Despite the side effects I listed, usually they are not a significant issue. Most side effects are mild and may resolve over time.

If the side effects are significant, though, most patients will not put up with them for long unless it's worth it. As we discuss the potential risks and benefits with each patient by observing the response to treatment, we can then tell if we are going in the right direction or if we need to change course. Once the patient and I are comfortable with the first step in order to build upon a solid foundation, then we can decide if we need to move on to the next step of augmentation.

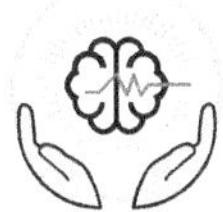

Dopamine and GABA/Glutamate
Part 1

Even though serotonin and/or norepinephrine are more often than not involved, there are some patients who do not respond well to an SSRI or an SNRI, and in those cases I shift my attention to dopamine and GABA/glutamate. For most patients I consider these two neurochemicals as secondary ones to address. However, the more uncommon patients in which serotonin and/or norepinephrine are not the issue are still seen frequently enough, and those cases need to be recognized so they can be treated properly. If the patient has bipolar disorder, then it may be best to address dopamine and/or GABA before addressing serotonin and/or norepinephrine. In bipolar spectrum patients, though, we often need to address 3 to 4 neurochemicals.

Whether to start with an antidepressant (which focuses on serotonin, norepinephrine, and/or dopamine) or a mood stabilizer (which focuses on dopamine and/or GABA/glutamate) depends on the presentation and history of the individual. Those with bipolar spectrum will most likely need to combine both classes. It really depends on which one to start with before augmenting with the other. If the patient is more in the depressed phase, then it is reasonable to start with an SSRI, an SNRI, or the NDRI Wellbutrin XL or the newer name-brand Aplenzin.

The newest antidepressant to come out in many years is the recently released, at the time of this writing, Auvelity (dextromethorphan/bupropion SR). It is a combination of Wellbutrin SR (which boosts dopamine as well as norepinephrine) with dextromethorphan, which boosts glutamate as well as slightly serotonin and norepinephrine. We have never seen such a unique mechanism of action that positively affects "The Fantastic Four" with one shot. I have heard from other doctors that they do not believe Wellbutrin XL augmentation is all that helpful, and they go straight for Auvelity (dextromethorphan/bupropion SR) instead. I don't understand how they cannot appreciate bupropion if they had any significant experience prescribing it. It is my top augmenting agent for a reason. If the Wellbutrin XL is increased to the maximum dose of 450 mg or Aplenzin to 522 mg, then I will probably reach for Auvelity (dextromethorphan/bupropion SR) samples. It is certainly nice to have so many excellent options to work with.

I also prescribe Lamictal (lamotrigine) for treatment-resistant depression, which actually means bipolar depression if it responds to Lamictal (lamotrigine). This is also the case if the depression responds to the atypical antipsychotic class whose main feature is dopamine antagonism as well as serotonin antagonism, which we will discuss next. If the patient presents in a hypomanic or manic fashion, it is probably safest and best to start with a mood stabilizer, and then after the mood is stabilized, consider adding an antidepressant.

If the patient has TRD (treatment-resistant depression), bipolar depression, or bipolar spectrum disorder, I would treat based on the current presentation and history and then make my best choice based on the evidence. If an antidepressant is chosen and lifts the patient out of depression but then leads to hypomania or mania symptoms, then the choice needs to be to either stop the antidepressant while attempting to stabilize the mood or to continue it to maintain the positive benefits while quickly adding a mood stabilizer to treat the residual symptoms of the upper pole. It depends on if the patient is getting adequate benefits from the antidepressants that would warrant the temporary instability and side effects, as long as the patient does not develop suicidal ideation because of the intervention. Since mood stabilizers act so quickly, the mania, hypomania, or high anxiety symptoms are usually able to be resolved quickly and adequately if the treatment is as aggressive as I need it to be. Otherwise, it may be better the first time to just stop the antidepressant and focus on stabilizing the mood first, since we can then make our decision about an antidepressant later. It really depends on the individual situation, since decisions are made based on the evidence and particulars. The rational polypharmaceutical approach requires the best combination of medications, whether they be antidepressants, mood stabilizers, stimulants, or other supplements.

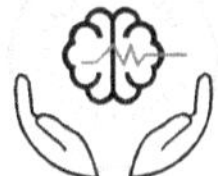

The Myth

A myth that has been perpetuated for far too long is that it takes 4 to 6 to 8 weeks for a psychotropic medication, especially an antidepressant, to start working. This myth has been perpetuated in every textbook that I have read on the subject, even the modern ones. I couldn't understand for years exactly why this myth has gone on for so long, but since I understand why now, I would like to try to debunk it and explain the truth of the subject. The reality is that most medications show efficacy within days to a week of starting them or after titration to the optimal dose, with the "acid test" being efficacious within two weeks. The quickest and most powerful medications, in a very good way. The GABA/glutamate agent Lamictal (lamotrigine) is the exception; it can take 3 to 4 weeks to start working and then possibly another 4 to 6 to 8 weeks to discover the optimal efficacy. I can tell you from experience that it is worth the wait. The quickest of the medications are also very fast-acting, working the same day, especially if the dose is right. Other augmenting agents also usually work very quickly, within a week or two being the usual measure of optimal efficacy.

I believe that this myth has been perpetuated since SSRIs have been the first-line treatment for over 30 years, since they may take weeks in order to titrate to achieve the ideal dose that provides the most efficacious results. A big problem I have seen is that doctors start at a low dose and titrate too slowly. If the titration is more aggressive, then the results should be realized quickly. If serotonin is the key neurochemical that is imbalanced, then the results are very quick, like the others, whereas if serotonin is only one of a combination of other neurochemicals imbalanced, then it will tend to work slower. If that is the case, then this hints at the fact that there is most likely a better psychotropic medication in a different class that will end up being a better choice for that individual.

SNRIs work more quickly simply because they do more by balancing two neurochemicals instead of one, and the response to balancing norepinephrine is very quick when it is optimally titrated. If an SSRI is either slow or leads to incomplete results, it is almost always a good idea to try an SNRI instead and compare and contrast the results. As I said before, these are usually the two neurochemicals that we start addressing when we first start treating mixed neurochemical imbalances with the rational polypharmaceutical approach.

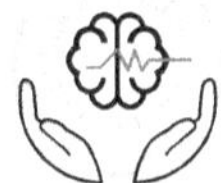

Dopamine - Part 2

Dopamine is certainly an interesting and exciting neuro-chemical to work with, given the impactful results and improved quality of life that result with dopaminergic agents. I refer to dopamine as the "pleasure chemical," since balancing dopamine properly by blocking its reuptake at the pre-synaptic cell membrane and thus increasing the dopamine level leads to improved motivation and drive, improved focus and concentration, lifting out of depression, improved energy, improved memory, an improved sex drive and sexual functioning, executive functioning, and improved functioning in general.

The medication that achieves all this is Wellbutrin XL (the form of bupropion I prescribe the most), which is in a class by itself, which now includes the newer name-brand version called Aplenzin. These are nDRIs, small n because it focuses more on dopamine and less on norepinephrine, though it is really a good combination of both. Wellbutrin is usually an augmenting agent that I add to an SSRI or an SNRI for unipolar disorder. An SNRI-Wellbutrin combination is my original "Dynamic Duo." For bipolar disorder, I may add it to an atypical dopamine antagonist and GABAergic agent, and it is often the ideal augmenting choice to achieve a boost out of the depths of depression, apathy, and fatigue. As I previously said, Auvelity (dextromethorphan/bupropion SR) also does what Wellbutrin does in the SR (sustained-release) form, with a component that also boosts glutamate as well as slightly serotonin and norepinephrine.

I call dopamine the "sex, drugs, and rock 'n roll" neuro-chemical, since dopamine is a key factor that is released when we experience certain pleasurable activities, which can drive some toward addictive behaviors to achieve in whichever way a pleasurable dopamine surge. Wellbutrin is one of the safest and more useful agents when it comes to bipolar depression, a critical component of bipolar disorder since those with this disorder spend far more time in depression than mania or hypomania. The most useful class of medication for mania and hypomania is dopamine antagonists; therefore, dopamine is the most key neurochemical when it comes to both poles of the bipolar spectrum. Since Wellbutrin is a medication that can dramatically improve the quality of life in some of our patients, it is important to be liberal with its use.

As I said, the other dopamine agents are the "atypical" antipsychotics, whose main purpose is as a dopamine antagonist (as well as a serotonin antagonist), which slows down and stops dopamine (and serotonin) when it's flying forward too quickly. When dopamine is going too fast, this can lead to mania, hypomania, insomnia, increased anxiety, increased depression, and increased anger and irritability. If the mind and thoughts are racing too fast, then this points toward the need to slow down dopamine. They are considered the "off" switch, while I consider Wellbutrin the "on" switch. I often use them together since they complement each other. In this way we can modulate dopamine by increasing its flow when needed and then decreasing and stopping its flow when appropriate.

If Wellbutrin improves mood and energy but increases anxiety or brings on hypomania or mania, then an atypical can be added to tune the person down. If an atypical works very well for the upper end of bipolar disorder but leads to depression, fatigue, and a flattening effect like apathy and low motivation, then adding Wellbutrin can quickly and reliably fix these problems. Sometimes the dose of the atypical needs to be increased when Wellbutrin is added in order to slow down dopamine properly when needed. When an atypical is increased to the ideal dose, this may lead to some sedation and other symptoms I just mentioned, due to dopamine moving too slowly in the daytime. Adding or increasing the Wellbutrin dose can easily fix this problem. The modern atypicals currently available are Risperdal (risperidone), Zyprexa (olanzapine), Seroquel (quetiapine), Seroquel XR (quetiapine ER), Abilify (aripiprazole), Geodon (ziprasidone), Invega (paliperidone), Fanapt (iloperidone), Saphris (asenapine), Latuda (lurasidone), Rexulti (brexpiprazole), Vraylar (cariprazine), Lybalvi (olanzapine and samidorphan), and Caplyta (lumateperone).

Though all of the atypicals are dopamine antagonists, which are also serotonin antagonists at the same time, some of them have partial dopamine agonism, which means most is pushed backwards while some is pushed forward, leading to less sedation, more energy, and improved cognitive functioning. This also seems to increase efficacy with overall fewer side effects. They also each have different effects on different parts of serotonin with antagonistic effects but also some with serotonin partial agonism, as well as some with beneficial effects on norepinephrine. All these different mechanisms of action come together to create excellent results while treating bipolar disorder, bipolar spectrum disorder, treatment-resistant depression, and other more difficult-to-treat variations of mood disorders. The atypicals are quick and excellent mood stabilizers that can help symptoms on both ends of the spectrum, which can lead to stability of mood over the long haul.

Lithium carbonate and Depakote are the "classic" mood stabilizers, though I use them far less than the atypicals. They may cause more side effects and require blood monitoring, ideally. They're still very useful, but due to the tolerance and efficacy of atypicals, this makes them tempting to use as first-line for mood stabilization. Lithium carbonate has been well-known to have positive effects when one is suicidal, but I believe all of the mood stabilizers and antidepressants can make the same claim, since optimally treating the underlying disorder dramatically reduces the risk of suicide. Even though I consider the atypical antipsychotics the first-line mood stabilizers, we should not forget about how impactful the "classic" mood stabilizers can be.

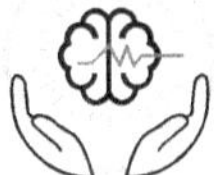

GABA/Glutamate - Part 2

GABA (gamma amino-butyric acid) and glutamate are the fourth of "The Fantastic Four" that I will now address. It is often one of the "forgotten" neurochemicals, along with norepinephrine and sometimes even dopamine, since serotonin attracts so much attention. When I speak of GABA, I'm also talking about glutamate, since they are opposites but complementary, in a sense opposite sides of the same coin.

Glutamate is the main excitatory neurochemical, while GABA is the main inhibitory neurochemical; thus, increasing GABA and/or decreasing glutamate leads to calming of the brain, while decreasing GABA and increasing glutamate leads to stimulation and excitation of the brain. I lump these "anti-seizure" medications together when I discuss GABA, though some of them do not directly affect GABA at all. However, I think of them all as GABAergic for the sake of simplicity.

The only "antidepressant" in this group is Lamictal (lamotrigine), and its main effect leads to suppression of glutamate with resultant calming of the brain as well as overall improvement of mood. Lamictal (lamotrigine) is an excellent medication for treatment-resistant depression, cyclical depression, or whichever variations of bipolar depression are more difficult to treat.

The GABA agents I usually prescribe are Topamax (topiramate), Neurontin (gabapentin), Depakote ER (divalproex sodium), and Lamictal (lamotrigine). I consider these mild mood stabilizers, though they are not all labeled as such. These work by improving the flow of GABA and/or suppressing the flow of glutamate, thus relaxing the brain, reducing anxiety, reducing hypomania and mania, improving sleep quality, resolving somatic symptoms, reducing cravings for certain foods, alcohol, and certain illicit drugs, and causing weight loss with some of them, such as Topamax (topiramate) and Keppra (levetiracetam), and potential weight gain with others, such as Depakote and Neurontin (gabapentin).

Topamax (topiramate) is, in my opinion, the best, least appreciated, and most underutilized medication in this class, and one that I prescribe very frequently, since it is unique and a very impactful medication. In addition to the above-listed benefits, it also helps patients lose weight. Wellbutrin is the only other psychotropic medication besides the name-brand Aplenzin and the newest antidepressant Auvelity (dextromethorphan/bupropion SR), along with a stimulant, of course. Topamax (topiramate) reduces cravings for sugars and carbohydrates, which drives down the intake of these foods along with the reduction of alcohol (liquid sugars and carbs) and sometimes even nicotine, marijuana, and other illicit drugs. It also makes sodas not taste the same by reducing their sensation of carbonation, which drives down their intake, which can be good since they're not good for us anyway. It also shares features of the other medications in this class, such as the reduction of somatic symptoms, reduction of headaches, reduction of anxiety, improved sleep, and overall improvement of mood. This is why I augment so often with this medication, since there is no other medication like it that does so much at one time.

It unfortunately has a bad reputation, with the nickname "Dopamax," since it has the potential to cause cognitive side effects. This fear is way overblown, though. In patients who would benefit from it, it is usually tolerated quite well if dosed slowly and carefully. It may take a week or two or more to realize the optimal dose, but it is worth the wait when it works. I typically have the patient take it mid-afternoon to early or later evening, at least an hour or so before the food cravings peak and when the increased eating starts. If they cannot remember the specific time, then I have them set an alarm on their phone to remind them. Starting at the lowest dose and titrating carefully over the first two weeks will reveal if the patient can tolerate it and if it works.

If the patient cannot remember to take it at this time, then it may be more convenient to switch to one of the longer-acting versions, Trokendi XR and Qudexy XR (both available in the generic form topiramate ER). The long-acting versions may be better tolerated and have better efficacy 24/7. They're also more convenient since they can be taken in the morning, while generic Topamax (topiramate) is often better when taken in the late afternoon to early evening, which can be difficult to remember for some. If it is not, though, the short-acting product can be taken twice a day. This is also a less expensive approach.

Neurontin (gabapentin) is another in this class that I use frequently, which is good for acute and chronic pain and acute and chronic anxiety and is a mild mood stabilizer, though it is not listed as such, as is the case with Topamax (topiramate). It can be very good for those who need to take a lot of benzodiazepines, since this can be substituted and has no addictive potential. It's quick-acting and short-acting like the benzodiazepines, so it can hopefully mimic the results. It can also help with sleep and restless leg syndrome, as is the case with the others in the class. Since fatigue, weight gain, and cognitive side effects are the main side effects, the dose may need to be lowered during the daytime and increased at night.

Depakote is also a very good medication in certain situations. It is effective for acute mania, hypomania, depression, anxiety, pain reduction such as headaches, and mood stabilization. It can be very good for certain bipolar patients who are more aggressive and have anger issues. The problem is that it may cause more side effects than others, such as fatigue and weight gain, and also needs blood monitoring. It is a good choice when atypicals are not adequately efficacious or are not tolerated. It also can be combined with atypicals for overall better efficacy, especially with the tougher bipolar patients. I have some experience with Trileptal (oxcarbazepine), Tegretol (carbamazepine), and Keppra (levetiracetam), though my experience with these is more limited. As I said, Topamax (topiramate) is by far and away the one I prescribe the most in this category, with Neurontin (gabapentin) and Lamictal (lamotrigine) in second and third place, with Depakote ER (divalproex sodium) coming in at fourth, with the others less frequently.

Lithium carbonate is one of the "classic" mood stabilizers, which reduces excitatory dopamine and glutamate but increases inhibitory GABA, which results in calming of the brain by achieving homeostasis. The other "classic" mood stabilizer, Depakote, works by increasing the transmission of GABA, which also has a calming effect on the brain. I don't prescribe these as often as the atypical antipsychotics, which I consider to be the first-line agents, though they are still extremely useful agents with the right individuals. For more difficult patients, combining different mood stabilizers from different classes, or two within the same class, such as combining two atypicals together, can be very effective to treat the most challenging cases.

There are other neurochemicals in the system besides "The Fantastic Four"—serotonin, norepinephrine, dopamine, and GABA/glutamate—that I will not be discussing in this book. The exception is Nuvigil (armodafinil), Provigil (modafinil), and Sunosi (solriamfetol), which boost not only dopamine but also, in the case of Nuvigil (armodafinil) and Provigil (modafinil), histamine, and in the case of Sunosi (solriamfetol), norepinephrine. This combination leads to the energizing effects seen with these medications. I discussed all of the medications that I have prescribed, along with details regarding dosage and titration of the medications, in the "Medication" chapters of my third book, which is mainly meant for doctors in my *Healing the Mind and Body* trilogy set.

Deplin (L-methylfolate) is a folic acid supplement, but it also increases the production of serotonin, norepinephrine, and dopamine, leading to antidepressant effects. It can be used on its own but is better when added to antidepressants. It can improve mood and energy, though it's still hit-or-miss.

Lastly, stimulants, which are most properly used for ADD/ADHD, also have a role in depression that may be more difficult to treat due to residual fatigue and depressive symptoms. Their action is to stimulate the forward flow of mostly dopamine but also norepinephrine, and they slightly bind to the receptors to prevent the reuptake of those chemicals. I will be discussing this class of medications later in this book, as well as all of the various psychotropic medications that we have the pleasure to work with.

Chapter One

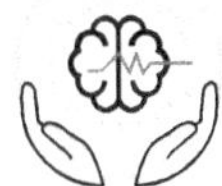

Conclusion

It is important to find the right mix of psychotropic medications and supplements for each patient in order to achieve the ultimate goal of full remission. It takes the rational poly-pharmaceutical approach in order to find the right cocktail for each individual. These answers are discovered along the way as we practice our techniques and witness the results for ourselves. This is the cutting edge of medicine today and in the future, since treating neurochemical imbalances so vastly improves the quality of life for our patients. The need is so great because this is the most underrecognized and under-treated public health crisis that is barely recognized. If the proper attention toward the subject became a reality, this would lead to a dramatic change in our society and world.

CHAPTER TWO

Depression

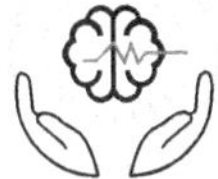

Depression

How do we define depression? This word means different things to different people. That's why I call it the "D word." Depression doesn't mean just being sad or "bummed out" occasionally. We all feel sad at times, and we all have good days and bad days. That's just a necessary part of the human condition. Clinical depression rather refers to a more pervasive and severe disorder, and it's vitally important that it is not ignored and is treated correctly. It could be a matter of life or death.

I'm going to now list some DSM-5 as well as some older DSM-IV "formal" diagnoses, and then I'll highlight some changes and updates in the newer DSM-5, which will highlight some of the evolving changes in thinking about depression over time. I will then give my more informal take on the subject. The field of medicine is always evolving, which is definitely the case in the field of mental health treatment, which I refer to as mind-body medicine. As we know more, we can learn and then change how we diagnose and treat these conditions in newer and better ways.

54

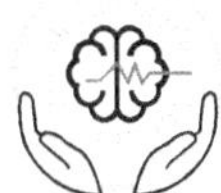

DSM-5 Definition of Major Depressive Disorder (MDD)

A. A mood disturbance described as follows:

Five (or more) of the following symptoms have been present for the same 2-week period and represent the change from previous functioning; at least one of the symptoms is either (1) depressed mood or (2) loss of interest or pleasure.

Note: Do not include symptoms that are clearly attributable to another medical condition.

1. Depressed mood most of the day, nearly every day, as indicated by subjective report (e.g., feels sad, empty, hopeless) or observation made by others (e.g., appears tearful). (**Note:** In children and adolescents, it can be an irritable mood.)

2. Markedly diminished interest or pleasure in all, or almost all, activities most of the day, nearly every

day (as indicated by either subjective account or observation).

3. Significant weight loss when not dieting or weight gain (e.g., a change of more than 5% of body weight in a month), or decrease or increase in appetite nearly every day. (**Note:** In children, consider failure to make expected weight gains.)

4. Insomnia or hypersomnia (sleeping too much) nearly every day.

5. Psychomotor agitation or retardation nearly every day (observable by others, not merely subjective feelings of restlessness or being slowed down).

6. Fatigue or loss of energy nearly every day.

7. Feelings of worthlessness or excessive or inappropriate guilt (which may be delusional) nearly every day (not merely self-reproach or guilt about being sick).

8. Diminished ability to think or to concentrate or indecisiveness, nearly every day (by subjective account or as observed by others).

9. Recurrent thoughts of death (not just fear of dying), recurrent suicidal ideation without a specific plan, or a suicide attempt or a specific plan for committing suicide.

B. The symptoms cause clinically significant distress or impairment in social, occupational, or other important areas of functioning.

C. The episode is not attributable to the physiological effects of a substance or to another medical condition. Note: Criteria A-C represent a major depressive disorder.

Note: Responses to a significant loss (e.g., bereavement, financial ruin, losses from a natural disaster, a serious medical illness or disability) may include the feelings of intense sadness, rumination about the loss, insomnia, poor appetite, and weight loss noted in Criterion A, which may resemble a depressive episode. Although such symptoms may be understandable or considered appropriate to the loss, the presence of a major depressive disorder in addition to the normal response to a significant loss should also be carefully considered. This decision inevitably requires the exercise of clinical judgment based on the individual's history and the cultural norms for the expression of the stress in the context of the loss.

D. The occurrence of the major depressive episode is not better explained by schizoaffective disorder, schizophrenia, schizophreniform disorder, delusional disorder, or other specified and unspecified schizophrenia spectrum and other psychotic disorders.

E. There has never been a manic episode or hypomanic episode, and criteria are not met for dysthymic disorder.

Note: This exclusion does not apply to all of the manic-like or hypomanic-like episodes that are substance-induced or are attributable to the physiological effects of another medical condition.

Specify:
- With anxious distress
- With mixed features
- With melancholic features
- With atypical features
- With mood-congruent psychotic features
- With mood-incongruent psychotic features
- With catatonia
- With peripartum onset
- With seasonal pattern (recurrent episode only)

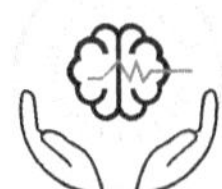

DSM-5 Definition of Minor Depressive Disorder

A. A mood disturbance described as follows:

1. At least two (but less than five) of the following symptoms had been present during the same 2-week period and represent a change from previous functioning; at least one of the symptoms is (a) or (b).

   (a) Depressed mood most of the day, nearly every day, as indicated by subjective report (e.g., feels sad, empty, hopeless) or observation made by others (e.g., appears tearful). (**Note:** In children and adolescents, it can be an irritable mood.)

   (b) Markedly diminished interest or pleasure in all, or almost all, activities most of the day, nearly every day (as indicated by either subjective account or observation made by others).

(c) Significant weight loss when not dieting or weight gain (e.g., a change of more than 5% of body weight in a month), or decrease or increase in appetite nearly every day. (**Note:** In children, consider failure to make expected weight gains.)

(d) Insomnia or hypersomnia nearly every day.

(e) Psychomotor agitation or retardation nearly every day (observable by others, not merely subjective feelings of restlessness or being slowed down).

(f) Fatigue or loss of energy nearly every day.

(g) Feelings of worthlessness or excessive or inappropriate guilt (which may be delusional) nearly every day (not merely self-reproach or guilt about being sick).

(h) Diminished ability to think or to concentrate or indecisiveness, nearly every day (by subjective account or as observed by others).

(i) Recurrent thoughts of death (not just fear of dying), recurrent suicidal ideation without a specific plan, or a suicide attempt or a specific plan for committing suicide.

2. The symptoms cause clinically significant distress or impairment in social, occupational, or other important areas of functioning.

3. The symptoms are not due to the direct physiological effects of a substance (e.g., a drug of abuse or a medication) or a general medical condition (e.g., hypothyroidism).

4. The symptoms are not better accounted for by bereavement (i.e., a normal reaction to the death of a loved one).

B. There has never been a major depressive episode, and criteria are not met for dysthymic disorder.

C. There has never been a manic episode, a mixed episode, or a hypomanic episode, and criteria are not met for cyclothymic disorder. **NOTE:** this exclusion does not apply if all of the manic-like, mixed-like, or hypomanic-like episodes are substance- or treatment-induced.

D. The mood disturbance does not occur exclusively during schizophrenia, schizophreniform disorder, schizoaffective disorder, delusional disorder, or psychotic disorder not otherwise specified.

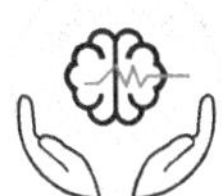

DSM-IV Diagnostic Criteria for Dysthymic Disorder

A. Depressed mood for most of the day, for more days than not, as indicated by subjective account or observation by others, for at least two years. **Note:** In children and adolescents, mood can be irritable, and duration must be at least one year.

B. Presence, while depressed, of two (or more) of the following:

(1) Poor appetite or overeating.

(2) Insomnia or hypersomnia.

(3) Low energy or fatigue.

(4) Low self-esteem.

(5) Poor concentration or difficulty making decisions.

(6) Feelings of hopelessness.

C. During the 2-year period (1 year for children or adolescents) of the disturbance, the person has never been without the symptoms in Criteria A and B for more than two months at a time.

D. No major depressive episode has been present during the first 2 years of the disturbance (1 year for children or adolescents); that is, the disturbance is not better accounted for by chronic major depressive disorder or major depressive disorder in partial remission.

Note: There may have been a previous major depressive episode, provided that there was a full remission (no significant signs or symptoms for 2 months) before development of the dysthymic disorder. In addition, after the initial 2 years (1 year in children or adolescents) of dysthymic disorder, there must be superimposed episodes of major depressive disorder, in which case both diagnoses may be given when the criteria are met for a major depressive disorder.

E. There has never been a manic episode, a mixed episode, or a hypomanic episode, and criteria have never been met for cyclothymic disorder.

F. The disturbance does not occur exclusively during the course of a chronic psychotic disorder, such as schizophrenia or delusional disorder.

G. The symptoms are not due to the direct physiological effects of a substance (e.g., a drug of abuse, a medication) or a general medical condition (e.g., hypothyroidism).

H. The symptoms cause clinically significant distress or impairment in social, occupational, or other important areas of functioning.

Specify if:

Early onset: if onset is before 21 years of age.
Late onset: if onset is at 21 years of age or older.

Specify if (for the most recent 2 years of dysthymic disorder):

With atypical features.

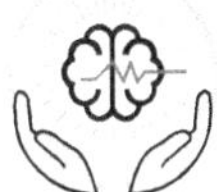

Depressive Disorder Due to Another Medical Condition

Certain medical conditions can lead to a state of depression, such as hypothyroidism, which can cause fatigue and weight gain and can also induce clinical depression. Among the criteria for this disorder is the level of disruption of normal activities like those related to one's occupation. Depression can be caused by a wide range of factors, and it is inherent in several medical illnesses, such as bipolar disorder. Yet a principle diagnostic characteristic of this type of depressive disorder is that it is not the result of some mental disorder; it is, instead, a consequence of medical conditions that are not always linked to depression.

Depression can stem from the fairly broad spectrum of medical conditions, from brain injury to Huntington's disease and Parkinson's disease. The correlation between a given medical condition and a depressive state varies in significance, but there is strong evidence that links depression with particular medical complications. The onset of this disorder differs depending on the medical condition under consideration. For example, depression usually occurs at the beginning of

Huntington's disease, and indeed, it is often the initial psychiatric condition of the disease.

Symptoms of depressive disorder due to another medical condition are contingent on the medical complication that the individual has. Broadly speaking, however, the depression symptoms are similar to those found in other depressive disorders, such as bipolar disorder and major depressive disorder. In seeking for symptoms of depressive disorder, the crucial step is to determine if the individual has a non-neuropsychiatric medical condition. As one of the symptoms that follow from this disorder, the DSM-5 notes that individuals with depressive disorder are not likely to find interest in many activities that were previously enjoyed, referred to as anhedonia, one of the two most sensitive and specific symptoms of depression. Additionally, if the mood disorder occurs when the patient does not have delirium, then a diagnosis of depressive disorder due to another medical condition may be warranted.

The DSM-5 criteria list some of the comorbid pathologies associated with depressive disorder due to another medical condition. There is considerable evidence that Parkinson's disease can induce a state of depression. At least 30% of Parkinson's disease patients have a depressive condition. Depression, however, is only one of many potential psychiatric symptoms, so attention toward this mind-body connection should be explored and adequately treated. Patients with Huntington's disease frequently have a depressive disorder of some kind, at least 50% of the time. The depressive symptoms of this disorder occur years before any motor symptoms of Huntington's disease are present, which can make it difficult to diagnose.

A CVA (cerebrovascular accident, a stroke) is often accompanied by depression, impacting 30% of stroke patients, making it the most common psychiatric disorder that follows the stroke. Patients with post-stroke depression are at a higher risk of mortality than post-stroke patients who have no depression. At least one in 10 cases of post-stroke depression report suicidal ideation, and hallmarks of post-stroke depression include social isolation and sleep complications. Other medical conditions that result in clinical depression have been briefly discussed by the DSM-5, which include Cushing's disease, brain injury, multiple sclerosis, and even sickle-cell anemia.

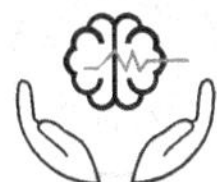

Substance- or Medication-Induced Depressive Disorder

The DSM-5 provides a complex and comprehensive iteration of substance-related disorders resulting from the use of a wide array of drugs, including tobacco, nicotine, alcohol, caffeine, marijuana, hallucinogens, opiates, inhalants, sedatives, or stimulants. Unknown substances may also trigger the disorder. Research points to the belief that substance-induced mood disorders (SIMDs) have been reported as early as the 1950s but may date back much further, to a time when psychiatry and medicine were in their infancy.

The DSM-5 explains that there are two separate types of substance-related disorders. There are those that are conditions of use and those that are induced with the abuse of substances. In the first case, the illness manifests with continued abuse in the face of presenting problems, while the latter opens the door to a wide variety of physical and psychological problems, including but not limited to psychosis, withdrawal, anxiety, and sexual dysfunction.

Substance/medication-induced depressive disorder has an array of associated comorbidities and risk presentations.

For example, individuals with a family history of depression, mood disorder, or substance abuse may be more inclined to suffer from this condition. Concurrent or associated problems may include a diagnosis of bipolar disorder, dysthymia, or depressive disorder. Substance/Medication-Induced Depressive Disorder has a variety of causes. Each case should be individually evaluated. It may be occurring due to the person's decision to abuse an illegal substance, or it may be the result of improper use of a medication that has been prescribed by a physician. It manifests itself in an equally extensive list of symptoms that include (but are not limited to) oversleeping, listlessness, social and emotional disengagement, sadness, suicidal thoughts, fatigue, a sense of hopelessness, and irritability. As this list indicates, there are a complex series of symptoms that may present differently in the case of substance/medication-induced depressive disorder. This disorder has an array of associated comorbidities and risk presentations. For example, individuals with a family history of depression, mood disorder, or substance abuse may be more inclined to suffer from this condition. Concurrent or associated problems may include a diagnosis of bipolar disorder, dysthymia, or depressive disorder.

Alcohol, substance, and/or medication dependency is in itself a depressing experience. It is characterized by relief that comes in the form of continued abuse and is a cycle that requires outside support to break. Even with adequate support, though, it can still be difficult to treat. Due to its insidious and often powerful but unexpected presentation in sufferers, the most realistic expectation is that the disorder be brought under control through a combination of medications, improved lifestyle habits, and psychological help. The team approach is often the most successful for many of the mind-body disorders.

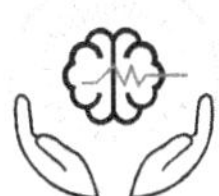

DSM-IV Diagnostic Criteria
for Depressive Disorder
Not Otherwise Specified

The depressive disorder not otherwise specified category includes disorders with depressive features that do not meet the criteria for Major Depressive Disorder, Dysthymic Disorder, Adjustment Disorder with depressed mood, or Adjustment Disorder with mixed anxiety and depressed mood. Sometimes depressive symptoms can present as part of an anxiety disorder not otherwise specified.

Examples of depressive disorder not otherwise specified include:

1. Premenstrual Dysphoric Disorder: In most menstrual cycles during the past year, symptoms (e.g., markedly depressed mood, marked anxiety, marked affective liability, and decreased interest in activities) regularly occurred during the last week of the luteal phase (and remitted within a few days of the onset

of menses). These symptoms must be severe enough to markedly interfere with work, school, or usual activities and must be entirely absent for at least one week post-menses.

2. Minor Depressive Disorder: episodes of at least 2 weeks of depressive symptoms but with fewer than the five items required for Major Depressive Disorder.

3. Recurrent Brief Depressive Disorder: depressive episodes lasting from two days to as long as two weeks, occurring at least once a month for twelve months (not associated with the menstrual cycle).

4. Postpsychotic Depressive Disorder of Schizophrenia: a major depressive episode that occurs during the residual phase of schizophrenia.

5. A major depressive episode superimposed on delusional disorder, psychotic disorder not otherwise specified, or the active phase of schizophrenia.

6. Situations in which the clinician has concluded that a depressive disorder is present but is unable to determine whether it is primary, due to a general medical condition, or substance-induced.

Discussion

Why do I list these older diagnoses? It's not just to bore you, but rather I want to highlight the differences with the newer "formal" criteria seen in the DSM-5. The newest

Diagnostic and Statistical Manual of Mental Disorders, 5th Edition (DSM-5), was released in 2013 and has a number of updates and changes made to major depression (also known as clinical depression) and depressive disorders. Dysthymic disorder, or dysthymia, is gone, replaced with something called "persistent depressive disorder." This new condition includes both chronic major depressive disorder and the previous dysthymic disorder. The reason for this change is that they were unable to find scientifically meaningful differences between these two conditions. Specifiers are used to identify different pathways to the diagnosis.

When it comes to clinical depression, formally known as major depressive disorder, the APA did not change the core criteria of symptoms for major depression, nor the requisite 2-week time period needed before it can be diagnosed.

The coexistence within a major depressive disorder of at least three manic symptoms (insufficient to satisfy criteria for a manic episode) is now acknowledged by the specifier "with mixed features." The presence of mixed features in an episode of major depressive disorder increases the likelihood that the illness exists within the bipolar spectrum. If the individual has never met criteria for a manic or hypomanic episode, the diagnosis of major depressive disorder is retained. Later in the Bipolar Disorder section I will be discussing in detail mixed episodes, mania, hypomania, and the whole bipolar spectrum.

The bereavement exclusion has been removed from the diagnosis of major depressive disorder in the DSM-5. This exclusion was only in effect if the person presented with major depressive symptoms within the first two months after the death of a loved one. This exclusion was omitted for several reasons. The first reason was to remove the implication that bereavement typically lasts only two months, while physicians and grief counselors recognize that the duration is more commonly one to two years. The second reason is that bereavement is recognized as a severe psychosocial stressor that can precipitate a major depressive episode in a vulnerable individual, generally beginning soon after the loss. When major depressive disorder occurs in the context of bereavement, it adds an additional risk for suffering, feelings of worthlessness, suicidal ideation, poorer somatic/physical health, worse interpersonal and work functioning, and an increased risk for persistent complex bereavement disorder, which is a new disorder listed in the DSM-5.

Major clinical depression related to bereavement is most likely to occur in individuals with past personal and family histories of major depressive episodes. It is genetically influenced and is associated with similar personality characteristics, patterns of comorbidity, and risks of chronicity and/or recurrence of major depressive episodes not related to bereavement. Although most people with bereavement experienced the loss of a loved one without developing a major depressive episode, evidence does not support the separation of the loss of a loved one from other stressors in terms of its likelihood of precipitating a major depressive episode with the relative likelihood that the symptoms will remit spontaneously.

Another reason I listed the older DSM-IV diagnoses was to show how similar they are to each other and how similar they are to the newer DSM-5 criteria of Major Depressive Disorder. No matter how we define depression, clinical depression is significant in whichever shape or form. Whether a person has 1 or 2 or 5 or more symptoms or whether it lasts 2 weeks, 2 months, or 2 years or more matters little to someone suffering. If a person is not feeling himself or herself and wants to get back to that normal and healthier state, then consideration should be given to treating it, whether it's minor, major, or in-between. As I said earlier, we all feel sad and bummed out at times, but clinical depression is more persistent and significant, and it can cause functional impairment as well as the risk of suicide. Clinically significant depression should never be ignored, no matter how major or minor.

When it comes to treating bereavement and adjustment disorder, it really depends on the specific needs of the individual, which can be determined based on history and clinical presentation. I don't believe that psychotropic medications interfere with the grieving process, so if the suffering causes significant impairment or difficulty functioning, then there is no reason not to treat it. These medications are not meant to blunt emotions but rather to help the person to be able to manage the grief and handle the stress. If there is no significant personal history of depression, then only a short trial of a psychotropic medication may be needed. It is also reasonable not to treat grief in certain people who may get through this difficult time with the support of family and friends and counseling when needed. It really just depends on the specific needs of the individual.

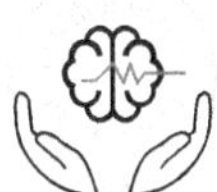

Other Depressive Mood Disorders

There are a couple of new diagnoses in the category of depressive disorders in the DSM-5: Disruptive Mood Dysregulation Disorder and Premenstrual Dysphoric Disorder. Disruptive Mood Dysregulation Disorder is a newly defined condition that addresses symptoms that had been labeled as "Childhood Bipolar Disorder" prior to the DSM-5. This new disorder can be diagnosed in children up to 18 years old who exhibit persistent irritability and frequent episodes of extreme, out-of-control behavior. I will list the formal criteria for the diagnosis, but the meaning and outcome are really the same. This likely represents early bipolar disorder or at least bipolar spectrum disorder that has not yet been diagnosed due to the age of the patient. I will discuss this issue more later on in the Bipolar Disorder section. I had already mentioned PMDD/PMS, which is newly defined as its own disorder in the DSM-5, so I will list the formal criteria. It is better known as PMS (premenstrual syndrome), though it is now more formally known as PMDD (premenstrual dysphoric disorder). It is common and quite easily treated. After these last two formal diagnoses are listed, I will then discuss my treatment approach for the depressive disorders.

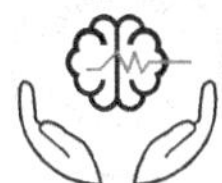

Disruptive Mood Dysregulation Disorder

The symptoms of DMDD go well beyond just temper tantrums. It is characterized by severe and recurrent temper outbursts that are grossly out of proportion in intensity or duration to the situation at hand. These occur, on average, three or more times each week for one year or more. Between outbursts, they display a persistently irritable or angry mood, most of the day and nearly every day, that is observable by parents, teachers, or peers. The diagnosis requires the symptoms be present in at least two settings (at home, at school, or with peers) for 12 or more months, and symptoms must be severe in at least one of these settings. During this period, the child must not have gone three or more consecutive months without symptoms. The onset of symptoms must be before the age of 10, and the diagnosis should not be made for the first time before age 6 or after age 18.

While prior to DSM-5 there were two diagnoses already with related symptoms to DMDD, Oppositional Defiant Disorder (ODD) and Bipolar Disorder (BD), the symptoms described in DMDD are different than these other two diagnoses. ODD is an ongoing pattern of anger-guided disobedience and hostilely defiant behavior toward authority figures that goes beyond the bounds of normal childhood behavior. While some of its symptoms overlap with the criteria for DMDD, the symptom threshold for DMDD is higher since the condition is considered more severe. It is now formally recommended that children who meet criteria for both ODD and DMDD should be diagnosed with DMDD.

BD also has similar symptoms; however, these children with DMDD may not present in an episodic way, as is the case with bipolar disorder. Children diagnosed with bipolar disorder who experience constant, rather than episodic, irritability are often at risk for major depressive disorder or generalized anxiety disorder later in life, but not necessarily lifelong bipolar disorder. In my opinion, though, probably many children with DMDD are on the bipolar spectrum, which I will discuss more later in this book.

This is important regarding not only diagnosis but also treatment, since if one is on the bipolar spectrum, then that individual may benefit from a combination of one or more antidepressants with one or more mood stabilizers. It is the same for DMDD. This severe of a presentation is not a unipolar disorder like MDD or anxiety disorder (which we will discuss in the next chapter). DMDD, in my opinion, is definitely early-onset bipolar disorder. I list it in this section because it is included with the depressive disorders in the DSM-5. There are many conditions and presentations that fall within the realm of the bipolar spectrum, which we will be discussing in chapter 4. As I said, the general rule of thumb is that the average patient on the bipolar spectrum is on about one to two antidepressants and one to two mood stabilizers. The higher-grade patients that spend more time at the upper pole will be on more mood stabilizers, while those who spend more time at the lower pole will likely need more antidepressants. Distinguishing between these disorders becomes very important when it comes to figuring out how to treat each person correctly.

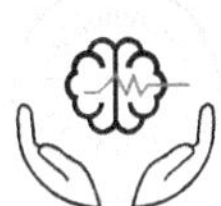

Premenstrual Dysphoric Disorder

PMDD is now an official diagnosis in the DSM-5. It is better known by the initials PMS (premenstrual syndrome), but now PMDD is considered the more technically correct diagnosis. In most menstrual cycles during the past year, five or more of the following symptoms occurred during the final week before the onset of menses, started to improve within a few days after the onset of menses, and were minimal or absent in the week post-menses, with at least one of the symptoms being either (1), (2), (3), or (4):

(1) Marked affective lability (e.g., mood swings; feeling suddenly sad or tearful or increased sensitivity to rejection).

(2) Marked irritability or anger or increased interpersonal conflicts.

(3) Markedly depressed mood, feelings of hopelessness, or self-deprecating thoughts.

(4) Marked anxiety, tension, and feelings of being "keyed up" or "on edge."

(5) Decreased interest in usual activities (e.g., work, school, friends, hobbies).

(6) Subjective sense of difficulty in concentration.

(7) Lethargy, easy fatigability, or marked lack of energy.

(8) Marked change in appetite, overeating, or specific food cravings.

(9) Hypersomnia or insomnia.

(10) A subjective sense of being overwhelmed or out of control.

(11) Other physical symptoms such as breast tenderness or swelling, joint or muscle pain, and the sensation of "bloating" or weight gain.

My purpose in listing these "formal" diagnoses is that it is important to try to define theoretically what we are treating clinically. However, it is even more important to understand that there are so many diagnoses that fall in-between the cracks that are all equally as important to recognize. For example, when it comes to major depression, minor depression, or dysthymia (depression-lite), the time frame of two weeks versus months versus two years or more is artificial, and all of the variations need to be treated anyway. Depression is depression and should be taken seriously no matter at what stage of whichever diagnosis. Whether one has one or two or more criteria versus five or more, that individual is suffering regardless, and that suffering needs to be attended to. What is striking to me is that there are no physical/somatic symptoms listed in the criteria for depressive disorders, other than PMDD. I am sure that you know by now how passionate I am about this subject. It is obvious that somatic symptoms relate to mood, and obviously there is a definite lack of recognition of this in these "formal" diagnoses. My hope is that my books will help to change the tide by sharing and speaking out about the theory and practice of the mind-body connection.

This is also the case for DMDD, ODD, and bipolar disorder, which are serious disorders that cause suffering not only for those who have them but also for those who have to deal with them.

For those who suffer with PMDD, whether they meet the criteria of five or more symptoms or less than five symptoms, this really doesn't matter much to the woman who suffers with it and still needs it attended to. Since there is so much interplay between formal diagnoses and informal diagnoses, this is why "off-label" treatment is even more important than "on-label" treatment, which should be the rule rather than the exception in my opinion. "Off-label" treatment is simply cutting-edge medicine at its best.

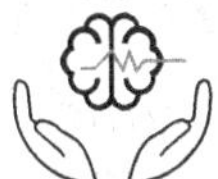

Treatment of Depression and Depressive Disorders

In order to determine the best treatment strategy, a full evaluation of the patient regarding a detailed history and symptoms is crucial. It is not always the case that medications are needed, though it is usually the case that proper psychotropic medications play an essential role. However, some may receive adequate treatment without medications, utilizing psychotherapy when needed. However, the evidence shows that psychotherapy and medications together lead to the best results. Other important factors are healthy lifestyle habits such as a regular exercise program and a well-balanced diet, learning coping skills, and learning how to relax with relaxation techniques, such as learning the low and slow breathing techniques, contemplative prayer, yoga, meditation, and others. A combination of these is often better than only one alone.

(1) **An SSRI versus an SNRI:** I don't mean to belabor the point, since I mention it so frequently, that it is more common to have both serotonin and norepinephrine

imbalanced at the same time rather than either one alone. I would guesstimate that at least 2/3 to 3/4 of patients have an imbalance of both instead of serotonin alone. Therefore, an SNRI is more often than an SSRI a better first-line choice as well as a choice to switch to after an SSRI is tried. It's reasonable to compare each class back-to-back if one is not sure which will be the better fit. SSRIs have been considered first-line medications for depressive disorders ever since the first one, Prozac (fluoxetine), came out. It may sound like it, but I am by no means anti-SSRI. They are excellent medications for the right person. I have prescribed them for many of my patients. However, I believe strongly that they are the best second-line agents, while SNRIs are the best first-line agents for the average individual more often than not.

I have seen many doctors switch patients from one SSRI to another, sometimes even four or five, before considering switching to another class. This drives me absolutely crazy, and it is a short drive. Doing the same thing over and over again and expecting a different result is the definition of insanity. For over 30 years I have considered SNRIs to be the overall best first-line choice, with SSRIs in second place. This truth that I discovered so long ago changed everything. Sometimes the best first-line choice is neither of these two, but rather a medication that addresses dopamine, GABA/glutamate, or both. I will discuss these more in a little bit.

How do we decide between an SSRI or an SNRI? It really just depends on the detailed history and review of symptoms. Serotonergic symptoms (related to an abnormal reuptake of serotonin in the nervous system) include symptoms of depression, anxiety-related symptoms, worry, rumination, obsessive thinking, PMDD, hormonally related symptoms, sexual symptoms (such as premature ejaculation and others), OCD, eating disorders such as anorexia and/or bulimia nervosa, insomnia (especially early-morning awakening), and others.

Noradrenergic symptoms (related to an imbalance of norepinephrine in the nervous system) are symptoms of depression, anxiety-related symptoms, and somatic/pain symptoms, including headaches; neck, shoulder, upper back, and lower back pain; TMJ syndrome; irritable bowel syndrome (IBS); fibromyalgia; joint pains; pain or discomfort in any area of the body; insomnia (difficulty getting to sleep and/or staying asleep); fatigue; poor focus and concentration; and others. Especially if anxiety and somatic symptoms are a part of the presentation, then more likely than not norepinephrine is in need of being balanced. If serotonergic symptoms predominate, then an SSRI may be the best first-line choice. However, if the patient has OCD, PMDD, or an eating disorder, an SNRI may still be better. Even though these conditions are usually mostly serotonergic, that does not mean that norepinephrine may not still be playing a role. This is where comparing and contrasting medications can be done to make sure the patient achieves the most complete results. It's difficult to tell fully based on just symptoms and history, since individuals respond in many different individual ways.

If an SSRI is picked, then it depends on how complete the results are and if there are any significant side effects. If the results are incomplete, even with proper titration and time, then it is reasonable to try switching to an SNRI rather than trying another SSRI. As I said before, way too many do this, which is usually a waste of time, and it also means that the patients continue to suffer needlessly. More often than not, the next correct choice is to try an SNRI. Sometimes the early results with an SSRI are very good, but then the efficacy decreases. If this does not respond to increasing the dose, or if it does but then the efficacy wears down again later, then this may be a good reason to change our approach. I frequently see the "SSRI Poop-Out Syndrome," which occurs only if serotonin is not the only neurochemical imbalanced.

Side effects related to SSRIs include fatigue, apathy, sexual side effects such as decreased interest, anorgasmia, delayed orgasm, and erectile dysfunction, activation/jitteriness, worsening of depression, worsening of anxiety, nausea, weight gain, and others. Even if the results of an SSRI after ideal titration are good, it's reasonable to switch to an SNRI to see if the results are even better. Why settle for good or even great if fantastic and excellent are achievable? It's worth the time it takes to make sure we get the first medication right before we consider moving on. Establishing the best possible foundation before proceeding, in my opinion, is essential.

If an SNRI is chosen first-line, second-line, or later, then we need to monitor what the positive results are and if any negative side effects are difficult to tolerate. Once the titration is complete, then we can consider whether to continue with it, switch to another in its class, switch to an SSRI, or try an antidepressant in a different class. SNRIs are less likely to "poop out" than the SSRIs, simply because they do more if more is needed. If noradrenergic side effects predominate, such as activation/jitteriness, dry mouth, nausea, constipation, urinary restriction, worsening of depression, worsening of anxiety, and potential insomnia. The SNRIs are less likely to cause sexual side effects and weight gain. If the side effects are mild, they may resolve over time, but if they are more severe and intolerable, they may still improve over time, but they also may not. If that is the case, this likely means that norepinephrine is fine and does not need any help. If the results are excellent and the side effects are minimal to none, then there may not be a reason to try an SSRI to compare with it. However, if an SSRI gives excellent results with no or minimal side effects, then the choice can be made as to whether to try an SNRI to see if it is even better or continue the same. It's very important to understand that if the results of one or the other are good, more than half the time the patient is still not in complete remission, which means that augmentation is usually required.

(2) **Wellbutrin** is an excellent augmentation strategy but also may be a first-line choice. Wellbutrin XL is by far the main form of bupropion that I prescribe, with the SR and IR versions much less common. Wellbutrin is really in a class by itself, with the newer name-brand bupropion XL available called Aplenzin. They are norepinephrine and dopamine reuptake inhibitors with a heavier effect on the dopamine and a lighter effect on the norepinephrine, which is why I label it as an nDRI. It is usually an augmenting agent that I add to an SNRI or an SSRI, but more rarely it is used as a primary antidepressant without the other two classes. If the patient does not do well with an SSRI or an SNRI with regard to either a lack of significant results, a predominance of side effects, or both, then this is a signal that neither of them are imbalanced and that it is time to look elsewhere for the answer. Dopamine is the next neurochemical that comes to mind.

Dopaminergic (and noradrenergic) symptoms related to an abnormal reuptake of both in the nervous system are fatigue, poor motivation and drive, lack of pleasure, poor focus and concentration (such as ADHD/ADD symptoms), decreased executive functioning, low sex drive or sexual functioning, decreased memory, decreased metabolism with weight gain, and desire to smoke cigarettes, as well as to use alcohol and illicit drugs.

If these symptoms predominate and there is a lack of significant symptoms related to serotonin or primarily nor-epinephrine, then it is reasonable to try Wellbutrin XL or Aplenzin as a first-line choice. If the results are good but incomplete, it is possible that serotonin and/or norepineph-rine are involved, even if less significantly so. If the results of Wellbutrin XL are good but side effects occur, such as anx-iety, depression, or other mood-related symptoms, then an SNRI or SSRI can be added to see if things balance out. It also may be possible that if Wellbutrin XL works but kicks up symptoms such as anxiety, irritability, insomnia, or others, then we may be dealing with one of the many types of bipolar disorders, which may need augmentation with a mood stabi-lizer rather than another antidepressant.

We are able to determine this based on a complete history and review of symptoms, whether we are more likely dealing with the spectrum of unipolar disorder versus the spectrum of bipolar disorder, or somewhere in-between the two spec-trums. Wellbutrin XL is also an excellent augmenting agent once other antidepressants and mood-stabilizing medications are already in place. If the results regarding mood are good, but if there is still residual depression, fatigue, lack of moti-vation, weight gain, poor focus and concentration (such as ADHD/ADD symptoms), if the patient is a smoker, lack of joy and pleasure, and others, then Wellbutrin XL may be the last piece of the puzzle that leads to full remission.

I have seen a trend of providers, including psychiatrists, not appreciating the role of bupropion as an augmenting agent.

I do not understand this thinking. Maybe many doctors do not have adequate experience prescribing this when augmenting with the primary agent? Maybe certain doctors don't appreciate the role of polypharmacy? Dopamine plays a very powerful and impactful role, and it concerns me that patients will not get into full remission unless the proper combination is given. I urge providers to gain more experience using this overall best augmenting agent that we have available.

(3) **Auvelity** (dextromethorphan/bupropion SR) is the newest antidepressant on the market, the only new one in several years, released in 2025, the same year that I completed this book. I have had several months of experience with it, and I am already quite impressed. It contains Wellbutrin SR, which focuses mostly on boosting dopamine but also secondarily boosting norepinephrine, while the dextromethorphan boosts glutamate and also slightly serotonin and norepinephrine. It is the only antidepressant that has ever been on the market that positively affects glutamate and the only antidepressant ever to have an effect on all of "The Fantastic Four." My approach, though, is to always augment with Wellbutrin XL first since it has an incredible track record. However, if it either doesn't work or works well but then "poops out" even when increasing it to the highest dose of Wellbutrin XL 450 mg or Aplenzin 522 mg, then it is time to move on. If that happens, I would probably reach for Auvelity (dextromethorphan/ bupropion SR) samples as my next choice. Even if the bupropion results are good, it doesn't hurt to try Auvelity (dextromethorphan/bupropion SR) and compare the two. Some of the doctors I mentioned above have shared that they bypass bupropion and jump straight

to Auvelity (dextromethorphan/bupropion SR). I vehemently disagree with this opinion.

(4) **Other choices.** There are other medications that help to balance dopamine besides bupropion XL. Nuvigil (armodafinil), Provigil (modafinil), and Sunosi (solriamfetol) are not stimulants but have stimulating effects. All three are primarily dopaminergic, but Nuvigil (armodafinil) and Provigil (modafinil) are also noradrenergic. Sunosi (solriamfetol) is the only noradrenergic. This is the only name-brand one on the market as a DNRI. The effect of having these neurochemicals boosted results in the energetic effects. We already know about norepinephrine and dopamine, but I don't mention histamine much. If we think of antihistamines as causing fatigue, if we do the opposite and boost histamine, it results in increased energy.

They are formally indicated for obstructive sleep apnea with resultant drowsiness as well as for shift workers who work the graveyard shift in order to increase energy during work hours. Nuvigil (armodafinil) and Provigil (modafinil) are generic, so the price has come down, though they are still not inexpensive. Sunosi (solriamfetol) came out in 2025, the year I finished this book. I have had results with this class of medications. Making them more affordable requires contacting the insurance company to do a prior authorization in order to try to get whichever medication approved on insurance. If you have experience in doing this, then it is simple enough to do.

(5) **The Atypicals:** Atypical antipsychotics focus primarily on dopamine and serotonin antagonism, with some possessing partial agonist properties at common dopamine and/or serotonin receptors and some with a slight norepinephrine effect. These are reserved more for bipolar depression, treatment-resistant depression, and other forms of depression that are more difficult to treat. They are typically augmenting agents, and very efficacious ones, but may be a solo agent for some.

I will be discussing this more in chapter 4, but I need to bring this up now because Rexulti (brexpiprazole) and Vraylar (cariprazine) are being marketed as augmenting agents to add to an antidepressant to treat MDD. This can be confusing, though, since it makes absolutely no sense that if we need to add an atypical antipsychotic to an antidepressant, we are dealing with MDD. It seems obvious that we are no longer in the unipolar realm but rather within the bipolar spectrum. Since most of bipolar disorder is spent in depression, it makes sense that a mood stabilizer would help. Even though I think it is false advertising, that is actually okay with me, as long as people are being helped. The reality is that most primary care providers are uncomfortable treating bipolar disorder and tend to refer to psychiatrists. As you know, I strongly believe that family physicians, internists, pediatricians, PAs, NPs, and other specialists of whichever area of medicine and others can prescribe. If the clinician gets the person better by adding an atypical and doesn't know exactly what they are treating, so be it. What matters most is that the patient gets better. For now, I am only mentioning Rexulti (brexpiprazole) and Vraylar (cariprazine), but I will list the other atypicals in chapter 4.

My hope is that the provider will eventually understand what they are really treating and become comfortable with treating the subtle and the more severe cases of bipolar disorder. I'm hoping that my books play a part in helping to make this happen.

(6) **Stimulants:** Other medications that stimulate the forward movement of dopamine and norepinephrine in the brain are the stimulants, such as ADD/ADHD medications and the weight loss drug Phentermine. These are very good choices if the patient has ADHD/ADD, but otherwise it depends on the situation. Some people tolerate them very well, while others may find them too harsh. Even though the main effect of stimulants is to stimulate the forward movement of the neurochemicals, especially norepinephrine and dopamine, they also slightly reduce the reuptake of both of them, which can lead to positive results with focus and energy as well as mood. They also cause a calming effect if one truly has ADD/ADHD. I consider a stimulant after I have already tried Wellbutrin XL, and if it is either not tolerated or tolerated well but there are still incompletely resolved symptoms such as fatigue, poor focus and concentration, poor memory, or poor metabolism, then switching or adding a stimulant is an option to consider.

We also need to consider the potential of addiction with certain patients. On the other hand, it may help the person to avoid the addictive drive if we treat the true underlying cause. Some people can't tolerate them, since they can cause too much anxiety, nervousness, jitteriness, insomnia, worsening of mood, or lowering of appetite. Stimulants are not my first-line choice unless the patient has ADD/ADHD; therefore, before trying a stimulant, I usually try at least a couple non-stimulants first.

(7) **Lamictal** (lamotrigine) is a unique antidepressant that is not meant for unipolar depression. It can be an excellent choice in certain situations. I consider it for more difficult-to-treat depression, such as treatment-resistant depression, bipolar depression, cyclical depression, and other in-between presentations that are really related to the bipolar spectrum. I consider it in the GABA/glutamate class when I list it among the other antiseizure medications such as Topamax (topiramate), Neurontin (gabapentin), Depakote ER (divalproex sodium), Trileptal (oxcarbazepine), and others, since most improve the forward flow of GABA within the nervous system. Others in this class, such as Lamictal (lamotrigine), actually have actions that result in the suppression of glutamate, the main excitatory neurochemical. This leads to a calming of the brain, which also occurs when a medication encourages the forward flow of GABA.

Lamictal (lamotrigine) is the slowest medication that I work with, but when it works, the results are amazing to see. Not only does it help pull the patient out of a tough depression, but it also prevents the patient from cycling back down into depression in the future. It can slow down or stop the cyclical nature of mood, even at times helping with bipolar mania and hypomania, though its focus is mostly on resolution of depression and its prevention in the future. This pattern can only be seen over time when one looks back and sees the course of the illness, with the goal being not only achieving complete remission but also staying there over the long haul. It can also be added to other antidepressants. The result can be very satisfying and can be the "last piece of the puzzle" that completes what we started, and it changes the long-term trajectory of the illness in a positive direction.

The other medications that I mentioned in this GABA class are more for anxiety reduction, somatic symptom reduction, weight loss, and stabilization of mood. When somatic symptoms are a part of the mood disorder, which is frequent, I think of norepinephrine first and GABA second and make sure that I attend to both when needed. I will discuss GABA further later when I discuss anxiety disorders in the next chapter. One is low in folic acid.

(8) **Deplin (L-methylfolate):** If the patient had a genetic mutation MTHFR, this results in poor metabolism of folate (folic acid). Deplin (L-methylfolate) is a high-quality L-methylfolate supplement. It is indicated, and when given to the right patient, it can increase the production of serotonin, norepinephrine, and dopamine. It can be tried as a solo agent for mild depression, but it's better as an augmenting agent to add to standard antidepressants.

(9) **Tricyclic antidepressants** are the other dual-action agents that balance serotonin and norepinephrine. I rarely prescribe them except for low doses as an augmenting agent for residual insomnia, anxiety, pain, or other somatic symptoms. The side effects at high doses tend to overpower the efficacy.

(10) **MAO inhibitors** are an option for more severe depression that hasn't resolved with other more standard anti-

depressants, such as the Emsam Patch (selegiline transdermal system) or one of the oral ones like phenylzine/Nardil. Even though I only rarely prescribe these, I've seen some very good results with some of these really tough patients, so it can certainly be worth a try. There are some dietary restrictions, but in reality, the vast majority of people don't need high quantities of these types of foods that would make this a danger, so the warnings are overblown. It is definitely a good class to consider if the other classes have been tried without success.

CHAPTER THREE

Anxiety Disorders

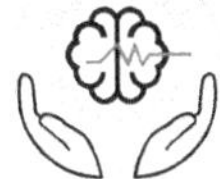

Anxiety Disorders

Anxiety is a normal human emotion. It is the response to specific types of stressful situations. Furthermore, not all the stressful situations that trigger anxiety are necessarily negative. The same is true for depression. All of us are sad at one time or another, but not everybody develops clinical depression. Anxiety disorders cross the line from regular stress and anxiety to a worsened and more persistent and pervasive problem that is important to treat.

Anxiety is a normal human emotion under circumstances of threat and is thought to be part of the evolutionary "fight or flight" reaction of survival. It is the response to specific types of stressful situations. It used to be a saber-tooth tiger attacking way back when, but now other modern equivalents lead to an abnormal amount of stress, which leads to anxiety that may get out of control. When it becomes maladaptive, then it leads to an assault on the mind and body that needs to be taken seriously.

Anxiety disorders are statistically the most common condition that I treat. Each year, anxiety disorders impact approximately 18%, or 40 million adults in the United States. Anxiety disorders have a lifetime prevalence of approximately 30%. Half of anxiety disorders at least also meet the criteria for a depressive disorder. Statistics are probably underestimated since most who have anxiety or another mood disorder often fail to be recognized and treated.

On the other hand, not all stressful situations that trigger anxiety are necessarily negative. Examples are a new and better job but new stress about performing, moving (even if it's a good move), having a baby, or anything that brings change. Stress often happens with a change of routine and pattern. Some people feel that stress drives them to perform better, while for others stress interferes with daily functioning. However we define it, stress is stress. We all experience it, so it really comes down to how much stress and one's ability to be able to cope with it. Stress refers to the tension exerted on a person, and stress arises from the distance between expectations and reality, obligation and resources, and current status and deadlines. The greater the distance, the greater the stress.

The core symptoms of anxiety are excessive fear and worry. Fear is the emotional response to real or perceived threats, whereas anxiety is anticipation of future threats. In comparison, the two key core symptoms of depressive disorders are depressed mood and loss of interest (anhedonia). Anxiety disorders and depressive disorders are very symbiotic and very often travel together. There is a lot of symptom overlap between the two disorders, such as sleep disturbance, fatigue, difficulty with focus and concentration, and others.

There is also a great deal of symptom overlap between the different anxiety disorders. In reality, anxiety disorders are frequently comorbid with many other conditions, such as ADHD, substance abuse, bipolar disorder, sleep disorders, and others. As with all the disorders I mention, there is a lot of variation between mild and more severe cases. This is why it's nice to have criteria, but if one falls below the criteria, that does not mean that person is suffering any less.

I will list the DSM-5 criteria for each of the main anxiety disorders, starting with the most common one, generalized anxiety disorder (GAD). You'll see a lot of overlap with, at times, subtle differences between them. You'll notice that they rarely list somatic/pain symptoms in the criteria, and you know my opinion about that by now. You will also notice that there are symptoms that overlap with not only depression but also other conditions, such as bipolar disorder and ADD/ADHD. It's certainly helpful to have formal criteria to go by and to have certain protocols, but in the end, it really comes down to how to best treat each individual, taking into account the whole person and all the details relating to that person.

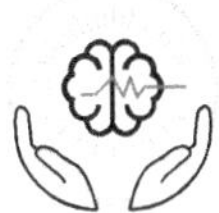

Generalized Anxiety Disorder (GAD)

Excessive worrying means worrying even when there is nothing wrong or in a manner that is disproportionate to the actual risk. This typically involves spending a high percentage of waking hours worrying about something. The worry may be accompanied by reassurance-seeking from others.

In adults, the worry can be about job responsibilities or performance, one's own health or the health of family members, financial matters, resolving conflicts, and other everyday, typical life circumstances. In children, the worry is more likely to be about their abilities or the quality of their performance, for example, in school.

- The worry experienced is very challenging to control.

- Worry in both adults and children may shift from one topic to another.

The anxiety and worry are associated with at least 3 of the following physical or cognitive symptoms (in children, only one symptom is necessary for a diagnosis of GAD):

- Edginess or restlessness.

- Tiring easily; more fatigued than usual.

- Impaired concentration or feeling as though the mind goes blank.

- Irritability (which may or may not be observable by others).

- Increased muscle aches or soreness.

- Difficulty sleeping (due to trouble falling asleep or staying asleep, restlessness at night, or unsatisfying sleep).

- Many individuals with GAD also experience symptoms such as sweating, nausea, or diarrhea.

- The anxiety, worry, or associated symptoms make it hard to carry out day-to-day activities and responsibilities. They may cause problems in relationships, at work, or in other important areas of one's life.

- These symptoms are unrelated to any other medical conditions and cannot be explained by the effect of substances, including prescription medication, alcohol, or recreational drugs.

- The symptoms are not better explained by a different mental disorder.

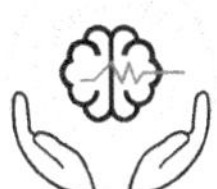

Social Anxiety Disorder (SAD)

The main feature of SAD is ongoing fear and worry surrounding a myriad of social situations. It is one of the most common mental disorders, with a lifetime prevalence of slightly greater than 10%. The majority of diagnoses are made during childhood or early adolescence. SAD often coexists with major depressive disorders, other anxiety disorders, and substance abuse disorders. Individuals with SAD often fear negative evaluation (e.g., being humiliated, embarrassed, or rejected) by others (either unfamiliar or familiar) in performance, interaction, or observation situations. Performance anxiety is the most common type and is actually the most common fear statistically. In the new DSM-5 criteria, children, adolescents, and adults all share the same criteria for duration, and the criterion for adult insight has been dropped.

SAD used to be called social phobia in the DSM-IV but has been renamed as social anxiety disorder. This change reflects a new and broader understanding of the condition in a variety of social situations. In the past, social phobia primarily was diagnosed in individuals who felt extreme discomfort or fear when performing in front of others. This definition is too narrow, though, as social anxiety can be diagnosed because of an individual's response to a variety of social situations. The person, for example, may be so uncomfortable carrying on a conversation that he is unable to talk to others, particularly someone he doesn't know. A person who is anxious over being observed may be unable to go out to dinner because she fears being watched while she is eating and drinking.

Social anxiety disorder is about more than just shyness, and it can be a considerably disabling condition. Diagnosis requires that a person's fear or anxiety be out of proportion, in either frequency and/or duration, to the actual situation. The symptoms must be persistent, lasting six months or longer. This time frame in the DSM-IV was only required for children, but this applies also to adults now. The minimum symptom requirement reduces the possibility that an individual's experience is only transient or temporary fear. To be diagnosed with SAD, the person must suffer significant distress or impairment that interferes with his or her ordinary routine in social settings, at work or at school, or during other everyday activities. Another update in the DSM-5 is that even if the individual has a lack of insight and does not recognize that his or her response is excessive or unreasonable, the criteria now shift that responsibility to the judgment of the clinician.

The clinician also needs to determine whether the person's reaction might be explained by such reasons as a more general anxiety or an adverse response to certain medications. If the person suffers from another medical condition (such as stuttering or obesity), the fear or anxiety experienced must be unrelated to the other condition or out of proportion to what would normally be felt. Several other criteria changes are specific to children to address social anxiety disorder at young ages. The DSM-IV includes severe, prolonged crying or tantrums, becoming physically immobilized, or shrinking away from other people. The DSM-5 includes extreme clinging and not being able to speak in social situations. These reactions can occur as a reaction to people the child knows or to strangers.

According to the DSM-5, there are a total of 10 diagnostic criteria for Social Anxiety Disorder:

1. Fear or anxiety specific to social settings, in which a person feels noticed, observed, or scrutinized. In an adult, this could include a first date, a job interview, meeting someone for the first time, delivering an oral presentation, or speaking in a class or meeting. In children, the phobic/avoidant behaviors must occur in settings with peers, rather than adult interactions, and will be expressed in terms of age-appropriate distress, such as clinging, crying, or otherwise displaying obvious fear or discomfort.

2. Typically, the individual will fear that they will display their anxiety and experience social rejection.

3. Social interaction will consistently provoke distress.

4. Social interactions are either avoided or painfully and reluctantly endured.

5. The fear and anxiety will be grossly disproportionate to the actual situation.

6. The fear, anxiety, or other signs of distress around social situations will be present for six months or longer.

7. The fear and anxiety caused personal distress and impairment of functioning in one or more domains, such as interpersonal or occupational functioning.

8. The fear, anxiety, or otherwise distressed situation cannot be attributed to a medical disorder, substance abuse, or adverse medication effects.

9. Fear or anxiety is not attributable to another mental disorder.

10. If another medical condition is present that may cause the individual to be excessively self-conscious (e.g., a prominent facial scar), the fear and anxiety are either unrelated or disproportionate. The clinician may also include the specifier that the social anxiety is performance-situation specific, such as oral presentations.

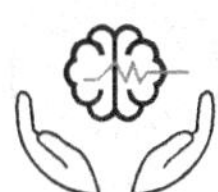

Post-traumatic Stress Disorder (PTSD)

In 2013, the American Psychiatric Association (APA) revised the PTSD diagnostic criteria in the DSM-5 over the years. It has introduced a preschool subtype of PTSD for children ages six years and younger. The criteria I will list below are specific to adults, adolescents, and children older than six years.

Diagnostic criteria for PTSD include a history of exposure to a traumatic event that meets specific stipulations and symptoms from each of four symptom clusters: intrusion, avoidance, negative alterations in cognition and mood, and alterations in arousal and reactivity. The fifth criterion concerns the duration of symptoms; the sixth assesses functioning; and the seventh criterion clarifies symptoms as not attributable to a substance or co-occurring medical condition.

Two specifications are noted, including delayed expression and a dissociative subtype of PTSD, the latter of which is new to the DSM-5. In both specifications, the full diagnostic criteria for PTSD must be met for application to be warranted.

Criterion A: Stressor

The person was exposed to death, threatened with death, suffered actual or threatened serious injury, or experienced actual or threatened sexual violence, as follows. (one required)

1. Direct exposure.

2. Witnessing, in person.

3. Indirectly, by learning that a close relative or close friend was exposed to trauma. If the event involved actual or threatened death, it must have been violent or accidental.

4. Repeated or extreme indirect exposure to aversive details of the event(s), usually in the course of professional duties (e.g., first responders collecting body parts; professionals repeatedly exposed to details of child abuse). This does not include indirect non-professional exposure through electronic media, television, movies, or pictures.

Criterion B: Intrusion Symptoms

The traumatic event is persistently re-experienced in the following way(s): (one required)

1. Recurrent, involuntary, and intrusive memories. **Note:** Children older than six may express this symptom in repetitive play.

2. Traumatic nightmares. **Note:** Children may have frightening dreams without content related to the trauma(s).

3. Dissociative reactions (e.g., flashbacks), which may occur on a continuum from brief episodes to complete loss of consciousness. **Note:** Children may reenact the event in play.

4. Intense or prolonged distress after exposure to traumatic reminders.

5. Marked physiologic reactivity after exposure to trauma-related stimuli.

Criterion C: Avoidance

Persistent, effortful avoidance of distressing trauma-related stimuli after the event. (one required)

1. Trauma-related thoughts or feelings.

2. Trauma-related external reminders (e.g., people, places, conversations, activities, objects, or situations).

Criterion D: Negative Alterations in Cognition and Mood

Negative alterations in cognition and mood that began or worsened after the traumatic event. (two required)

1. Inability to recall key features of the traumatic event (usually dissociative amnesia; not due to head injury, alcohol, or drugs).

2. Persistent (and often distorted) negative beliefs and expressions about oneself or the world (e.g., "I am bad," "The world is completely dangerous").

3. Persistent distorted blame of self or others for causing the traumatic event or for resulting consequences.

4. Persistent negative trauma-related emotions (e.g., fear, horror, anger, guilt, or shame).

5. Markedly diminished interest in (pre-traumatic) significant activities.

6. Feeling alienated from others (e.g., detachment or estrangement).

7. Constricted affect: Persistent inability to experience positive emotions.

Criterion E: Alterations in Arousal and Reactivity

Trauma-related alterations in arousal and reactivity that began or worsened after the traumatic event. (two required)

1. Irritable or aggressive behavior.

2. Self-destructive or reckless behavior.

3. Hypervigilance.

4. Exaggerated startle response.

5. Problems in concentration.

6. Sleep disturbance.

Criterion F: Duration

Persistence of symptoms (in criteria B, C, D, and E) for more than one month.

Criterion G: Functional Significance

Significant symptom-related distress or functional impairment (e.g., social, occupational).

Criterion H: Exclusion

The disturbance is not due to medication, substance abuse, or other illness.

Specify if with dissociative symptoms.

In addition to meeting criteria for diagnosis, an individual experiences high levels of either of the following in reaction to trauma-related stimuli:

1. **Depersonalization:** Experience of being an outside observer of or detached from oneself (e.g., feeling as if "this is not happening to me" or as if one were in a dream).

2. **Derealization:** Experience of unreality, distance, or distortion (e.g., "things are not real").

Specify if with delayed expression.

A full diagnosis is not met until at least six months after the trauma(s), although onset of symptoms may occur immediately.

Post-traumatic Stress Disorder (PTSD) is included in a new chapter in the DSM-5 on Trauma and Stress-Related Disorders. This more addresses PTSD as an anxiety disorder, which is one of several changes approved for this condition, which is increasingly at the center of public as well as professional discussion.

The diagnostic criteria for the manual's next edition identify the trigger to PTSD as exposure to actual or threatened death, serious injury, or sexual violation. The exposure must result from one or more of the following scenarios, in which the individual:

1. Directly experiences the traumatic event.

2. Witnesses the traumatic event in person.

3. Learns that the traumatic event occurred to a close family member or close friend (with the

actual or threatened death being either violent or accidental).

4. Experiences firsthand repeated or extreme exposure to aversive details of the traumatic event (not through media, pictures, television, or movies unless work-related).

The disturbance, regardless of its trigger, causes clinically significant distress or impairment in individuals, in social interactions, capacity to work, or other important areas of functioning. It is not the physiological result of another medical condition, medication, drugs, or alcohol.

The DSM-5 draws a clear line when detailing what constitutes a traumatic event. Sexual assault is specifically included, for example, as is a recurring exposure that could apply to police officers or first responders. Language stipulating an individual's response to the event, such as intense fear, helplessness, or poor coping, has been deleted because that criterion proved to have no utility in predicting the onset of PTSD. The DSM-5 also paid more attention to the behavioral symptoms that accompany PTSD and proposes four distinct diagnostic clusters instead of three. They are described as re-experiencing, avoidance, negative cognition and mood, and arousal.

Re-experiencing covers spontaneous memories of the traumatic event, recurrent dreams related to it, flashbacks, or other intense or prolonged psychological distress. Avoidance refers to distressing memories, thoughts, feelings, or external reminders of the event.

Negative cognition and mood represent feelings, from a persistent and distorted sense of blame of self and others to estrangement from others or markedly diminished interest in activities or to an inability to remember key aspects of the event.

Finally, arousal is marked by aggressive, reckless, or self-destructive behavior, sleep disturbances, hypervigilance, or related problems. The DSM-5 emphasizes the "flight" aspect associated with PTSD as well as the "fight" reaction often seen.

The number of symptoms that must be identified depends on the cluster. DSM-5 only requires that the disturbance continue for more than a month and would eliminate the distinction between acute and chronic phases of PTSD.

The DSM-5 includes the addition of two subtypes: PTSD in children younger than six years and PTSD with prominent dissociative symptoms (either experiences feeling detached from one's own mind or body or experiences in which the world seems unreal, dreamlike, or distorted).

There is debate in the military about PTSD. Certain military leaders, both active and retired, believe the word "disorder" makes many soldiers who are experiencing PTSD symptoms reluctant to ask for help. They may feel that this is a weakness in their character and goes against the "macho" image a soldier wants to convey. They have urged the change to rename the disorder post-traumatic stress injury, a description that they say is more in line with the language of troops and would reduce stigma. Others, however, believe that the military environment needs to change, not the name of the disorder, so that mental health care is more accessible and soldiers are encouraged to seek it out in a timelier fashion. Some were concerned that "injury" is too imprecise a word for a medical diagnosis.

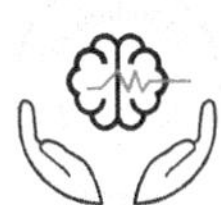

Agoraphobia

Agoraphobia is newly defined as an anxiety disorder in the DSM-5. It represents an intense fear resulting from real or imagined exposure to a wide range of situations. It is most commonly known as people who have a fear of public places. An essential feature is the fear of situations where the escape from the perceived bad things may be difficult. Those who have agoraphobia disorder experience significant and persistent fear when in the presence of, or anticipating the presence of, at least two situations. These situations may include crowds, public places, public transportation, being outside of the home, open spaces, standing in line, being isolated, and over-dependence. To meet the new DSM-5 criteria, when in these situations, the person must engage in avoidance behaviors to avoid the fear and/or a related panic attack. Further DSM-5 criteria for this disorder are:

- Marked and out-of-proportion fear of the presence or anticipation of a specific situation.

- Exposure to the phobic stimulus provokes an immediate anxiety response, which may then take the form of a situationally bound or situationally predisposed panic attack.

- The person recognizes that the fear is out of proportion.

- The phobic situation(s) is avoided or else is endured with intense anxiety or distress.

- The avoidance, anxious anticipation, or distress in the feared situation(s) interferes significantly with the person's normal routine, occupational (or academic) functioning, social activities, or relationships, or there is marked distress about having the phobia.

- The symptoms of agoraphobia for all ages must have a duration of at least six months.

- The anxiety, panic attack, or phobic avoidance associated with the specific situation is not better accounted for by another mental disorder.

- Many of the physical symptoms of agoraphobia are also experienced in a panic attack and include nausea, dizziness, sweating, rapid heart rate, stomach upset, chest pains, and diarrhea.

Under DSM-5, several changes have been made to prevent the overdiagnosis of agoraphobia based on the overestimation of danger or occasional fears. A person no longer has to demonstrate excessive or unreasonable anxiety for a diagnosis of agoraphobia. Instead, the anxiety must be "out of proportion" to the threat considering the environment and situation. Psychotherapy plus medications often leads to the best results for all the anxiety disorders and other mood disorders mentioned in this book.

Agoraphobia can have a severe impact on the daily life of those who suffer with it, some of whom had become famous recluses, such as Howard Hughes. The level of social interaction may also be predicted by whether or not the agoraphobic has panic attacks, a disorder very closely related to agoraphobia. Those with panic attacks tend to withdraw more from society than those who don't have them. Others may avoid uncomfortable situations and make mild to moderate accommodations to their lives. In addition to medications, psychotherapy such as CBT (cognitive behavioral therapy) can be very helpful, and now with modern technology it can be done in a "safe" environment of one's home.

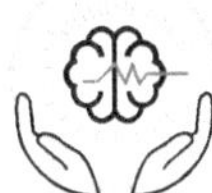

Obsessive-Compulsive Disorder (OCD)

The diagnosis of OCD in the DSM-5 must meet both the general and the specific characteristics of this disorder and must meet these general criteria:

- You must have obsessions and compulsions.

- The obsessions and compulsions must significantly impact your life.

- You may or may not realize that your obsessions and compulsions are excessive or unreasonable.

Your obsessions must meet specific criteria:

- Intrusive, repetitive, and persistent thoughts, urges, or images that cause distress. It may feel as if one has lost his or her mind.

- The thoughts do not just excessively focus on real problems in your life.

- You unsuccessfully tried to suppress or ignore the disturbing thoughts, urges, or images.

- You may or may not know that your mind simply generates these thoughts and that they do not pose a true threat.

Your compulsions must meet specific criteria:

- Excessive and repetitive ritualistic behavior that you feel you must perform, or something bad will happen. Examples include hand washing, counting, silent mental rituals, checking door locks, etc.

- The ritualistic compulsions take up at least one hour or more per day.

- You perform these physical rituals or mental acts to reduce the severe anxiety caused by the obsessive thoughts.

Clinicians face some challenges in making an obsessive-compulsive disorder diagnosis, since the symptoms can appear similar to those with an anxiety disorder, clinical depression, schizophrenia, and a number of other mental illnesses. Some drugs or other medical conditions can also mimic the symptoms of OCD, so it's up to the clinician to make the appropriate diagnosis. Treatments such as medications and psychotherapy are very effective, so many people with the disorder can lead productive and happy lives.

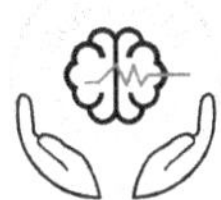

Separation Anxiety Disorder

An individual with SAD (not to be confused with social anxiety disorder) displays anxiety and fear atypical for his or her age and development level over separation from people and places to which he or she has a strong attachment. Two important changes were made to Separation Anxiety Disorder in the DSM-5. It is no longer a disorder that only has its onset in childhood. There is no specified age of onset now. It is now characterized under anxiety disorders rather than disorders usually first diagnosed in infancy, childhood, or adolescence. It is now recognized that SAD also can develop in adulthood. Victims of war and natural disasters of any age may experience SAD. War veterans experience SAD, often comorbid with PTSD. SAD is a predictor of psychopathology in adulthood, as it can develop into other disorders such as panic disorder, major depressive disorder, and agoraphobia.

Separation anxiety is normal in children until about 3 to 4 years of age. Some children continue to experience significant anxiety and stress over separation and may display social withdrawal, as well as having difficulties sleeping and at school. A child raised in a very close family may be more prone to acquire the disorder. The child may also display higher fears toward the unknown when separated from an attachment figure.

He or she may fear physical harm and death to himself or herself as well as loved ones. Negative emotions may include anger and feelings of neglect. Stress-related physical symptoms can also develop, such as nausea, headache, stomach ache, palpitations, and vomiting. Those with adult separation anxiety disorder (ASAD) who have also experienced early separation anxiety are more likely to have other anxiety disorders, including avoidant, dependent, and obsessive-compulsive disorder. The majority of people with SAD also have clinical depression.

The DSM-5 criteria for Separation Anxiety Disorder are:

SAD must persist in individuals under 18 for at least four weeks and adults for six months or more. An individual with SAD experiences persistent anxiety at a developmentally abnormal level in response to separation or impending separation from an attachment figure, as evidenced by three of the following symptoms:

- Recurrent obsessive stress when anticipating or experiencing separation from major attachment figures or home.

- Persistent and excessive worry about losing major attachment figures or harm to them.

In response to fear of separation from an attachment figure:

- Excessive worry about experiencing a negative event (e.g., an accident or illness, being lost or kidnapped).

- Refusal to go out, such as from home, to school, or to work.

- Fear of being alone without major attachment figures at home or in other settings.

- Reluctance or refusal to sleep away from home or to go to sleep.

- Repeated nightmares involving the theme of separation.

- Repeated complaints of physical symptoms when separation of major attachment figures occurs or is anticipated.

For a diagnosis of separation anxiety disorder, the individual must experience a clinically significant level of distress or impairment in social, academic, occupational, and other areas of functioning that is not explained by another disorder. Children with autism, for example, often do not respond to social cues, but their social deficits are unrelated to detachment disorder. For example, the person with agoraphobia may have a fear of going outside, and panic attacks are also associated with SAD.

A child with separation anxiety may refuse to attend social events, such as a visit to a friend's house, or attend school. A child may engage in oppositional behaviors such as temper tantrums, screaming, crying, and hitting. Oppositional behavior is often the most pronounced toward going to school, but this does not always qualify as SAD. Agoraphobia could also be behind the defiant behavior. School refusal may also be related to low grades or bullying. Homesickness is also a natural experience for most children. Early identification and proper diagnosis are important in order to ensure early treatment and thus better treatment outcomes. Some with SAD may manifest delinquent behavior at a later stage in life, including school delinquency and substance abuse and dependence. As in other anxiety disorders, CBT and/or medications can be very effective.

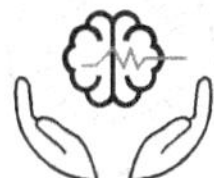

Panic Disorder

Panic disorder is defined as recurrent, unexpected panic attacks. Panic attacks are abrupt surges of intense fear or discomfort that occur abruptly and peak rapidly. A panic attack is a discrete period of intense fear or discomfort emerging either from a calm or anxious state; they can either be expected or can come "out of the blue" and can happen when one is active or at rest. In my experience, though, I have seen that this usually happens when one is at rest, even when trying to wind down at the end of the day after work. This is when one's guard is down, and then the anxiety can emerge. These rarely occur when one is exercising or otherwise active. When this happens, I encourage patients to practice their slow breathing exercises, or another remedy is to go out and take a quick walk or jog or do another type of active exercise.

They occur abruptly and peak rapidly. They can happen with several other mental and medical problems. We will focus now, though, on panic disorder, and the essential features are persistent fear or concern of inappropriate fear responses with recurrent and unexpected panic attacks with associated physiological changes such as accelerated heart rate, sweating, dizziness, trembling, chest pain, and others. Panic disorder has physical and cognitive symptoms and involves numerous, unexpected panic attacks, though some are expected too.

Panic attacks occur in over 11% of the general population, and about 2 to 3% of the general population has panic disorder. The median age of onset ranges between 20 and 24 years old, more or less. A smaller percentage is first diagnosed in childhood and is not usually first seen over the age of 45. Public speaking is statistically the #1 fear, even more than the fear of death. Isn't that interesting? People are more afraid to speak in front of others than to die? Illness anxiety disorder, formerly known as hypochondriasis, often shares features with and/or is comorbid with panic disorder.

According to the DSM-5, the most prominent diagnostic criterion for panic disorder is recurrent unexpected panic attacks. Because the panic attacks are unexpected, they may be impossible to predict and come out of nowhere. This surge of fear can occur when the person is already anxious, or it can occur during a calm state when a person is relaxing, sleeping, or even engaging in an enjoyable activity. Common features of panic attacks include an accelerated heart rate or pounding heartbeats, chest pain or chest pressure, shortness of breath, hyperventilating, holding one's breath, sweating, shaking, trembling, the choking sensation, nausea, dizziness or lightheadedness, numbness, tingling, chills, increased heart rate, sweating, feeling of being detached from oneself or losing control, fear of dying, etc. In addition to panic attacks, the patient experiences persistent worry or fear of having a panic attack and often changes behaviors and routines to avoid these panic attacks. People who experience unexpected panic attacks often become fearful of experiencing one at work, with friends, or in public. They're concerned that they may be judged for their behavior or lose control and are fearful of being embarrassed. It's important to make sure that the symptoms are not related to substance use or abuse or other medical or psychiatric conditions.

The formal DSM-5 diagnostic criteria for panic disorder include previous diagnoses from the DSM-IV of panic disorder with and without agoraphobia, and the symptoms include:

A. Recurrent unexpected panic attacks.

B. At least one of the attacks has been followed by 1 month (or more) of one or both of the following:

1. Persistent concern or worry about additional panic attacks or their consequences (e.g., losing control, having a heart attack, going crazy).

2. Significant maladaptive change in behavior related to the attacks (e.g., behaviors designed to avoid having panic attacks, such as avoidance of exercise or unfamiliar situations).

C. The panic attacks are not restricted to the direct physiological effects of a substance (e.g., a drug of abuse, a medication) or a general medical condition (e.g., hyperthyroidism, cardiopulmonary disorders).

D. The panic attacks are not restricted to the symptoms of another mental disorder, such as social phobia (e.g., in response to feared social situations), specific phobia (e.g., in response to a circumscribed phobic object or situation), obsessive-compulsive disorder (e.g., in response to dirt in someone with an obsession about contamination), post-traumatic stress disorder (e.g., in response to stimuli associated with a traumatic event), or separation anxiety disorder (e.g., in response to being away from home or close relatives).

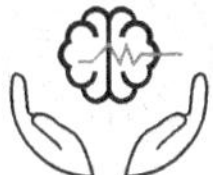

Anxiety Disorder Due to Another Medical Condition

In this condition, the most frequently displayed symptom is anxiety in some form, even though there is another medical condition present that underlies and leads to the anxiety. On review, the symptoms can include palpitations, sweating, muscle tension, dizziness, shortness of breath, racing heart, and many others that I have previously listed. In addition to these physical symptoms, anxiety also can lead to restlessness, a fear of impending doom or catastrophe, or a fear of being embarrassed or humiliated. If the anxiety leads to panic disorder, symptoms can include a sudden onset of terror with no specific precipitating event, leading to a racing and pounding heart, sweating, dizziness, or feeling faint. If the symptoms also include nausea, numbness of the hands and arms, chest pressure or pain, and difficulty breathing, the patient may think that he or she is suffering a heart attack and call 911 or go to the ER. This fear of impending doom and feeling of losing control can increase the anxiety and panic and thus worsen the symptoms.

If the anxiety is rather experienced as generalized anxiety disorder (GAD), the individual may feel generalized worry and tension with little or no precipitating event. They may feel a sense of impending doom or disaster regarding work, home life, financial status, or general health. They have difficulty relaxing, have an exaggerated startle response, and have difficulty focusing and concentrating. GAD can also present with physical symptoms such as headaches, muscle tension, gastrointestinal symptoms, irritability, being quick to anger, fatigue, difficulty breathing, nausea, sweating, lightheadedness, etc. If the anxiety presents as OCD, there are intrusive thoughts that bring on anxiety that are not within that person's control. This leads the person to perform certain rituals and behaviors that temporarily decrease the anxiety, and the rituals can then control the person's behavior. Checking and rechecking things, touching objects in a certain order, and counting are among the most common rituals. The thoughts that trigger anxiety may have to do with harming loved ones, performing sexual acts that are otherwise unacceptable to the person, or thinking about things that go against the person's religious beliefs.

In order to qualify for this diagnosis, no matter how the anxiety is exhibited, it must be due to the direct physiological effects of another medical condition and can parallel the course of the illness. It is thus important to get a thorough history, perform a complete physical exam, and obtain appropriate labs and other diagnostic studies in order to establish this direct effect between the physical and emotional. This diagnosis can be made if it is not better explained by another mental disorder and does not occur only during the course of delirium. Clinically significant distress must be present, and the functioning of the person in social, occupational, or other areas of life must be impaired. A thorough medical evaluation is needed to determine the presence of the medical condition that leads to the anxiety. Some of the medical conditions that may be involved in this disorder are hypothyroidism, hyper-thyroidism, and other endocrine disorders and heart-related problems such as congestive heart failure and cardiac arrhyth-mias. Breathing problems such as COPD, asthma, pneumonia, and hyperventilation can also increase anxiety, along with many neurological conditions. There must be a close associa-tion between the medical condition and the anxiety in order to meet this diagnosis. The anxiety symptoms must occur close in time to the onset, worsening, or lessening of the med-ical condition. If the features of anxiety are not typical for a primary anxiety disorder, and there is a medical condition present whose physiological effects contribute to the anxi-ety, then this is an indication that "Anxiety Due to Another Medical Condition" may be the appropriate diagnosis.

As I already said, to make this diagnosis, the anxiety should not occur just during the course of delirium. However, it is appropriate to make the diagnosis if the anxiety occurs directly due to dementia. It is also important to differenti-ate anxiety due to the effects of continuing substance use or abuse, along with withdrawal from a substance or exposure to a toxic substance, which would lead to a diagnosis of sub-stance-induced anxiety. A thorough medical evaluation and drug screens are useful in this situation. It is also possible to have a dual diagnosis of anxiety due to another medical condition and substance-induced anxiety disorder if criteria for both diagnoses are met. This condition also should be dif-ferentiated from another primary anxiety disorder, as I said, or from an adjustment disorder. In another primary anxiety disorder, there is no direct link to a medical condition that causes the anxiety.

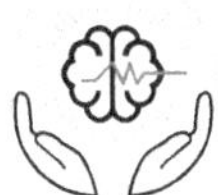

Substance- or Medication-Induced Anxiety Disorder

The DSM-5 diagnostic criteria for substance/medication-induced anxiety disorders are those of the other anxiety disorders, primarily anxiety and panic. Obsessions and compulsions should not be present, as in obsessive-compulsive disorder, which may also be precipitated by drugs or medications, and now have their own category. Symptoms must develop during or within a month of use or intoxication, or within a month after withdrawal from a drug or substance known to cause anxiety. It must not be ascribable to other anxiety disorders and must not be the result of delirium caused by the drug. The responsible drug or drugs should be identified.

This disorder is characterized by anxiety or fear, sometimes accompanied by physical symptoms such as racing heart, shortness of breath, shakiness, nervousness, and others, caused by the effects of the medication or psychoactive substance. Although "anxiety" and "fear" are often used interchangeably, the former generally means an unpleasant emotional state for which the cause is not apparent or which is perceived to be uncontrollable, while the latter is usually the emotional and physical response to an unidentifiable threat. Another way of putting it is that anxiety is the anticipation of future events, while fear is a reaction to current events.

These symptoms may occur while the patient is under the influence of the drug (intoxication) or after the use of the drug has stopped (withdrawal). Generalized anxiety or panic attacks were manifestations of phobias that may be precipitated by either substance use or withdrawal. Obsessions and compulsions were formally considered anxious manifestations of substance use but are now categorized separately as substance- or medication-induced obsessive-compulsive disorder.

Anxiety caused by the drug may persist as long as use continues, while withdrawal-related symptoms may first manifest themselves up to four weeks after cessation of use. Prolonged psychiatric symptoms, including anxiety and panic, can continue for up to six months and have rarely been reported four years after cessation of alcohol, benzodiazepines, opioids, and even occasionally antidepressants. This is a signal, though, that we may be dealing with a bipolar variant that should be explored.

Alcohol, amphetamines, methamphetamines, cannabis, cocaine, PCP, hallucinogens, and others have been reported to cause symptoms of anxiety during intoxication. Withdrawal from alcohol, cocaine, nicotine, caffeine, and others can also manifest as anxiety. Many prescription and even over-the-counter medications can cause anxiety, including common cold medications, excessive thyroid supplementation, cardiac medications, asthma medications, and even antidepressants and mood stabilizers. It's really individualized because certain people are just extra sensitive to certain substances.

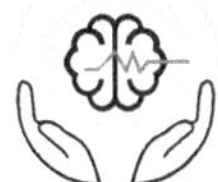

Hypochondriasis

Hypochondriasis has been redefined in the DSM-5, with sweeping changes in the category of somatoform disorders. In the DSM-5, hypochondriasis and related conditions have been replaced by two new diagnostic concepts: illness anxiety disorder and somatic symptom disorder. They differ markedly from the somatoform disorders in DSM-IV.

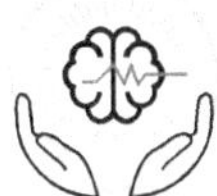

Illness Anxiety Disorder

Patients with illness anxiety disorder may or may not have a medical condition but have heightened bodily sensations, are intensely anxious about the possibility of an undiagnosed illness, or devote excessive time and energy to health concerns, often obsessively researching them. They are not easily reassured even when presented with scientific evidence. Illness anxiety disorder can cause considerable distress and disruption of one's life due to obsessiveness that borders on the irrational.

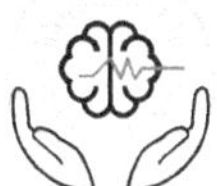

Somatic Symptom Disorder

Patients with somatic symptom disorder have one or more chronic somatic symptoms about which they are excessively concerned, preoccupied, or fearful. These fears and behaviors cause significant distress and dysfunction in life. Even when patients frequently use health care services, they are rarely reassured and often feel that their medical care has been inadequate, leading to "doctor shopping" in a futile search for answers to their satisfaction.

Some feel that these new diagnoses are overly broad and likely to lead to increased mental health diagnoses in the medically ill. I would argue the opposite, and I'm happy that somatic symptoms are finally getting the recognition they deserve as having an important role in the diagnosis of anxiety-related illnesses. There is a significant under-diagnosis of relevant mental health diagnoses due to the lack of recognition of how frequently somatic symptoms relate to stress and mood. Hopefully these new diagnoses will help to increase the recognition of how frequently these mind-body conditions occur. Those who have reasonable health concerns do not qualify for these diagnoses. Those with unexplained symptoms that are being worked up may be justifiably a little anxious until the results are known. It can become abnormal, though, if patients are abnormally preoccupied beyond reason, when a complete and reasonable workup reveals no significant abnormalities, or even if real medical conditions occur but result in an abnormal preoccupation, worry, and fear beyond reason.

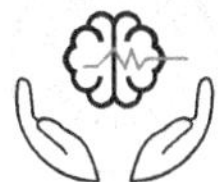

Illness Anxiety Disorder (IAD)

According to the new DSM-5 criteria, the symptoms of IAD include:

1) Preoccupation with the idea that one has or will get a serious illness.

2) Lack of somatic symptoms, or mild somatic symptoms, such as diaphoresis or slight tachycardia.

3) If there is a verifiable medical condition present (e.g., a benign cyst), or the patient is in a high-risk category for developing a medical condition (e.g., heart disease), but there are no current indicators of heart disease. The patient's anxiety or concern is out of proportion to the objective reality.

4) The patient is hyper-vigilant about his or her health and is prone to feeling distressed about their health, changes in their health, or ambiguous symptoms.

5) The patient will frequently monitor themselves for signs of illness, such as checking their blood pressure or temperature several times a day.

6) The patient will avoid medical care or evaluation due to anxiety about what they imagine will be found.

7) This anxiety and preoccupation will have persisted at least six months, although the source of anxiety will shift (e.g., fear of diabetes will be superseded by fear of cancer).

8) The anxiety and preoccupation with illness are not better accounted for by another mental disorder, including somatic symptom disorder, panic disorder, GAD, OCD, or a psychotic episode with somatic delusions.

The clinician can add specifiers to the diagnosis:

- **Care-seeking type:** The patient will frequently seek medical care, presenting with health concerns and complaints, and undergoing diagnostic procedures.

- **Care-avoidant type:** The patients will have anxiety about presenting themselves for diagnosis and avoid medical care.

Other components of the clinical presentation of IAD can include:

- Frequent, dramatic statements regarding one's health.

- Self-pity.

- Exaggeration of the impact or actual disorders.

- Dramatic response and preoccupation with minor injuries.

- Claiming to have unverifiable disorders or a disorder persisting for an implausible length of time.

- Lack of response and reassurance from medical providers.

A thorough medical work-up, sometimes exhaustive testing, and consultation with specialists will fail to yield any objective evidence of serious medical problems. The basis of the patient's distress is anxiety about a misinterpretation of a physical symptom or sign. If there is a verifiable condition, it needs to be minor, easily treated, benign, and self-limiting; the result of normal function; or within normal limits of uncomfortable sensations that do not indicate illness.

The patient may not only have anxiety about health and disease in themselves but also in people around them. They may react strongly to news of medical conditions such as the 2014 Ebola epidemic in West Africa. They may project their health-related anxiety onto family members, overreacting to minor illnesses or injuries in children. IAD can lead people to limit their lifestyle and activities, and they may adopt an imagined disease as their primary identity. People with IAD may thrive on attention and sympathy. They tend to discuss and complain about their health excessively, causing discomfort in others, eventually causing others to avoid them, resulting in social constriction or isolation. The ironic risk is that if the person with IAD truly becomes ill, people around them may not respond, or they may be isolated to the extent that they have no one to respond to them, like in the fable *The Boy Who Cried Wolf.*

They may have difficulty accepting the diagnosis of a psychological disorder, as they are convinced there is something medically wrong with them, and they may feel their concerns are being discounted. It is noted that people with hypochondriasis may have rigidly held beliefs and convictions about their health that are not supported by scientific evidence.

An individual with IAD may research the disease(s) they imagine they have, sometimes inducing what is commonly referred to as "Medical Student Syndrome." This refers to the erroneous belief that one has a medical condition, based on incomplete knowledge or "too much" knowledge, as they may not have the context to understand the conditions they are studying. An example of this is the current trend of gluten-free foods. Celiac disease, or gluten intolerance, is a genuine, verifiable medical condition, but many will self-diagnose and then adopt the restricted diet based on the belief they have this disorder. Misattribution of apparent benefits may emerge partly due to a placebo effect.

Individuals with IAD tend to overutilize healthcare services, have extensive medical care, invasive diagnostic procedures, and sometimes unneeded elective surgery. They may crave the attention and care they get. Being the center of attention of a team of highly trained and skilled individuals can be rewarding to them. They may have multiple providers and can frustrate care providers, who may not be as thorough as they are accustomed to due to groundless complaints from the patient. Iatrogenic disease can result from complications due to invasive diagnostic and testing procedures.

According to the DSM-5, IAD often begins in early to middle adulthood and may be a lifelong condition. A personal or family history of serious or chronic illness or an experience with the medical profession that diminished one's faith, trust, or confidence in physicians can lead to IAD. It may be set off by a major stressor or a serious but eventually benign threat to the individual's health. Child abuse or serious illness in childhood can perpetuate IAD in an adult.

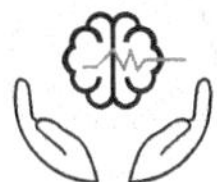

Differential Diagnosis for Illness Anxiety Disorder

The DSM-5 describes the following rule-out diagnoses for the clinician to consider:

- Other legitimate medical conditions: One can really be sick and still have IAD. The non-medical provider must have the collaboration of the medical team to rule out legitimate conditions. IAD indicates that the response to an actual illness is out of proportion to the severity of the illness.

- Adjustment Disorder.

- Health-related anxiety is a non-pathological response to a serious illness.

- Somatic Symptom Disorder is the appropriate diagnosis when there are significant somatic symptoms. In contrast, individuals with IAD (Illness Anxiety Disorder) have minimal or absent somatic symptoms, but their primary concern is that they have an illness.

- Anxiety Disorders, including GAD: The anxiety will stem from multiple sources, which could include their health, but health will not be the primary focus. Individuals with panic disorder may be hypersensitive to respiratory or cardiac symptoms that may be benign.

- Body Dysmorphic Disorder: The individual will be focused on an imagined flaw in her or his appearance.

- Major Depressive Disorder: People who are depressed can have somatic symptoms (e.g., headaches, stomach aches, muscle and joint pain, and the reduced tolerance for discomfort) and the possibility of mood-congruent delusions. The preoccupation will be limited to the acute depressive episode.

Other considerations for differential diagnosis include:

- Munchhausen Syndrome: Deliberate induction of the medical disorder for secondary psychological gains (e.g., attention from medical staff).

- Malingering: The possibility that the patient is feigning illness for secondary gains must be considered.

- Drug seeking: Patients present themselves at ERs and PCPs' (primary care physicians') offices seeking opiates or benzodiazepines to sustain their addiction. This is also known as "doctor shopping," in which an opiate or benzodiazepine addict will visit numerous physicians or ERs, complaining of non-verifiable conditions to obtain drugs. This is distinct from IAD, in that the motive is to obtain abusable drugs, and they do not believe they have an illness that requires medication. However, opiate addicts are specifically hypersensitive to signals from their bodies that are reminiscent of withdrawal symptoms.

Approximately two-thirds of individuals with IAD are likely to have at least one other comorbid form of psychopathology:

- Somatic Symptom Disorder: This disorder involves some degree of physical symptoms, which have a psychological basis.

- OCD can either be comorbid with IAD, or IAD may be a form of OCD. Some individuals with IAD experience intrusive images, including the diagnosis of a terminal illness, suffering with it, dying, and the aftermath of their death for their family. OCD has neurological commonalities with IAD.

- GAD (Generalized Anxiety Disorder): The content of anxiety can include it but will not be limited to health concerns. This is a rule-out as well as a potential comorbidity.

- PTSD: Trauma content can center on physical concerns, e.g., someone with a recent MI (myocardial infarction) may overreact to innocuous and ambiguous chest discomfort.

- Psychosis: Somatic delusions will have bizarre content and no basis in reality.

- BPD (Borderline Personality Disorder): Dramatic complaints about physical symptoms from minor injuries, or fabrication or even induction of a disorder (Munchhausen syndrome) can occur as part of the borderline presentation.

- Histrionic Personality Disorder: Part of the dramatic presentation can include greatly exaggerated or frequent complaints of medical problems or an overly emotional response to a minor injury.

- Orthorexia: Exclusion of certain foods without sufficient objective evidence or formal diagnosis (e.g., gluten intolerance).

- Exacerbation of serious medical conditions due to avoidance of medical care or such frequent presentation for medical care that providers do not take legitimate complaints seriously.

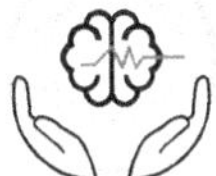

Somatic Symptom Disorder

This condition also recognizes the prominence of somatic symptoms associated with significant emotional distress and impairment. Individuals who have disorders with prominent somatic symptoms are often encountered in the primary care office, in the office of specialists, in the emergency room or urgent care centers, and in the offices of psychiatrists, as well as therapists, social workers, pharmacists, and other providers that deal with these patients. As is the case with illness anxiety disorder, this is a reconceptualized diagnosis that has replaced the diagnosis of somatoform disorder in the DSM-IV. I welcome this new category of somatic symptoms and related disorders, since this just goes to show how important the interplay is between mental and physical health, the mind-body connection. I'm excited about the fact that the importance of this topic is becoming more recognized and more accepted.

Somatic symptom disorder (SSD) is characterized by somatic symptoms that are either very distressing or result in significant disruption of functioning, as well as excessive and disproportionate thoughts, feelings, and behaviors regarding those symptoms. To be diagnosed with SSD, the individual must be persistently symptomatic for at least six months. This diagnosis replaces the previous DSM-IV diagnoses of hypochondriasis, somatization disorder, pain disorder, and undifferentiated somatoform disorder. In the DSM-IV, the diagnosis of somatization disorder required a specific number of complaints from among four symptom groups, among them neurological symptoms, gastrointestinal symptoms, and sexual or reproductive symptoms. The SSD diagnosis does not have such a requirement; however, the somatic symptoms must be significantly distressing or disruptive to daily life and must be accompanied by excessive thoughts, feelings, or behaviors.

Medically unexplained symptoms are the key feature for many of the somatic disorders in the DSM-IV, but in the DSM-5, to meet a diagnosis of SSD does not require that the somatic symptoms be medically unexplained. In other words, symptoms may or may not be associated with another medical condition. This points to the idea that it is not appropriate to diagnose individuals with a mental disorder solely because the medical cause cannot be demonstrated. Whether or not the somatic symptoms are medically explained, in order to meet the diagnostic criteria for SSD, the rest of the criteria would still need to be met. The good news is that this new diagnosis is simpler than the combination of somatic disorders previously recognized.

The vast majority of these patients are typically seen in a primary care setting and not in the psychiatric practices, so it's important for primary care providers to recognize the link between physical symptoms and emotion. It's also very important for psychiatrists to learn to recognize that somatic symptoms play an important role in the overall presentation of many patients that they see. Psychiatrists may not learn adequately about the physical body and the role of somatic symptoms in order to fully understand the mind-body connection.

However, the mind and body cannot be separated, one necessarily affecting the other. This recognition can then lead to better treatment strategies that are currently often employed.

It is vitally important that primary care providers, psychiatrists, and other specialists perform a comprehensive assessment of patients in order to recognize that psychiatric problems often coexist with medical problems. Instead, the DSM-IV focuses on medically unexplained symptoms, while the DSM-5 rather emphasizes the degree to which a patient's thoughts, feelings, and behaviors about their somatic symptoms are disproportionate or excessive. Some patients with real physical conditions such as heart disease or cancer may still experience disproportionate and excessive thoughts, feelings, and behaviors related to their illness, and some of them qualify for a diagnosis of SSD. Just as depression and anxiety can occur in the context of a medical disorder, so can this diagnosis. It is thus important to recognize when a patient's thoughts, feelings, and behaviors are indicative of a mental disorder that can then be diagnosed and treated appropriately. It is difficult to separate the mind and body, since both just happen to be the same individual.

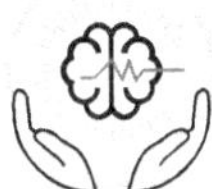

Treatment of Anxiety and Somatic Disorders

In order to determine the best treatment strategy, a full evaluation of the patient regarding history and symptoms is crucial. Psychotropic medications are usually very effective, but there are non-medication approaches that can also help, at times by themselves but more often with medications. Psychotherapy can be effective, and it has been shown that medications plus psychotherapy is more effective than either alone, as is the case with depression. Healthy lifestyle habits are very important for complete treatment, since a regular cardiovascular exercise program can really help to decrease anxiety and stress. Coping strategies are also important in order to learn how to deal with stress. Relaxation techniques such as breathing techniques, yoga, meditation, and contemplative prayer can also be invaluable.

Regarding treatment for anxiety disorders and somatic disorders, you will notice some similarities and differences as compared to treatment of depression. In reality more than half the people with anxiety disorder also have depression and vice versa. Depressive disorders are sometimes viewed as "anxious misery" with high incidences of sadness and anhedonia. Anxiety disorders often include "anxious anticipation," uncertainty, and fear. Sleep disturbance, fatigue, difficulty with concentration, and other symptoms can be symptoms of both. As I said before, I list the "formal" diagnoses in order to highlight not only the differences but also the similarities between different types of mood disorders. For more information about anxiety and stress, check out the second book of the *Healing the Mind and Body* trilogy series, chapter 3, "Managing Stress," and chapter 4, "Anxiety Disorders."

1) **An SSRI versus an SNRI:** I don't mean to belabor the point, but this is a crucial decision. I'm trying to not repeat myself too much, so for more details go to this section on the treatment of depression disorders earlier in the book. This is usually the first decision when treating both anxiety and depression, and it's important to get the first step right. The majority of anxiety and somatic disorders involve the neurochemical imbalance of serotonin and/or norepinephrine, more often both than either alone. I would guesstimate that at least two-thirds to three-quarters of the time an SNRI is a better and more complete choice than an SSRI. This is also the case with depression and depressive disorders but is even more likely to be true for anxiety and somatic disorders. Earlier in this book, I reviewed symptoms that I feel are more serotonergic and others that I feel are more noradrenergic, but it is difficult to separate that out since there is so much overlap.

SSRIs are less complete when it comes to treating somatic symptoms and anxiety symptoms, so even if an SSRI is being taken and works fairly well, it is still worthwhile to try an SNRI to see if even better results are within our reach, since we have so many good choices. Norepinephrine is one of the two key neurochemicals that I consider addressing when somatic and anxiety symptoms are present, along with GABA, which I will discuss next. I typically address norepinephrine first, however, with an SNRI before I consider augmenting.

If neither an SNRI nor an SSRI provides excellent results without significant side effects, which, as I said, is not usual, then I move on to consider GABA first and then probably dopamine next, or possibly the other way around depending on the situation. It's very important to get the first step right before we move on to the second step, since it is easier to build on a good foundation. The goal of the first medication is to provide the best possible results with the least or no side effects. Even with an SNRI, though, more than half of people with anxiety or somatic disorders are not in full remission, which is why augmentation is so important and is the norm rather than the exception.

2) **A GABAergic medication:** GABA is often the second most significant neurochemical in need of being imbalanced when we deal with anxiety and somatic disorders, or it might be first. These medications usually improve the forward flow of GABA from neuron to neuron, and since GABA is the main inhibitory neurochemical, this leads to a calming effect on the body and mind. Some rather inhibit the release of glutamate, which is the main excitatory neurochemical, which also leads to calming of the brain and rest of the body.

My two favorite medications to prescribe in this class are Topamax (topiramate) in the short-acting or one of the longer-acting forms and Neurontin (gabapentin), in that order. Topamax (topiramate) is one of my favorite augmenting agents to prescribe since it is so unique and so useful. It not only reduces anxiety and somatic symptoms but also helps patients lose weight if they need to, which is unusual among psychotropic agents. It mainly reduces the desire for sugars and carbohydrates, thus decreasing the impulse to indulge in "stress eating" and "comfort foods." (The only other two medications that help to promote weight loss are Wellbutrin and stimulants, but those can increase anxiety for some).

Topamax (topiramate) is best known for the prevention of migraine headaches, but it also helps for the prevention of many other somatic symptoms. The most significant side effect to watch for is cognitive side effects, though for most it is not an issue if titrated and dosed correctly. The options currently available are generic Topamax (topiramate) and topiramate ER (also available in their long-acting brand names Trokendi XR and Qudexy XR).

Neurontin (gabapentin) is my second favorite in this class, and it is also very effective for somatic and anxiety symptoms. It is well known and prescribed not only by primary care doctors and psychiatrists but also neurologists and pain specialists and is used for a variety of disorders. Some examples are neuropathic pain, peripheral neuropathy, severe pain syndromes such as trigeminal neuralgia and restless leg syndrome, and a variety of neurological and pain disorders. It also is very useful for anxiety disorders and for those addicted to tranquilizers, even those on high doses of benzodiazepines, which can be very addictive, since Neurontin (gabapentin) is quick-acting and can be dosed multiple times per day, as can be the case with the benzos. We need to monitor for fatigue and cognitive side effects, as is the case with Topamax (topiramate). It can also help people who are addicted to opiates. It does not lead to weight loss, as is the case with Topamax (topiramate), and can rather lead to weight gain. In these situations, I often add Topamax (topiramate), and it is very safe and effective to combine these two together, as is the case with the other GABA agents that can lead to weight gain, such as Depakote ER (divalproex sodium). It is an invaluable medication in this important medication class.

The other class of medications that I just mentioned that also temporarily balance GABA are the benzodiazepines (minor tranquilizers), such as Xanax (alprazolam), Klonopin (clonazepam), Ativan (lorazepam), Valium (diazepam), Librium (chlordiazepoxide hydrochloride), and others. Their main action is their tranquilizing effect and quick resolution of anxiety, even with anxiety attacks and panic attacks, but the other effect is quickly moving GABA forward through the nervous system, leading to the calming effect. The problem with them is that they can work *too well* and thus be *too easy* to take, even for milder anxiety that may get better with relaxation techniques and exercise. They certainly have significant addictive potential, especially when not used properly, which is only as needed for more moderate to severe anxiety. There is no question that they are very effective and useful agents to combat the miserable symptoms of acute anxiety; however, I try to minimize the use of the "quick fix" agents like these in favor of more preventative medications like Topamax (topiramate), Neurontin (gabapentin), and the others in this class. It's best for our patients to minimize the "Band-Aid" solutions and maximize the preventative and curative solutions instead, such as psychotropic medications. We need to get under the hood and treat the core underlying problems, rather than dealing with them after the fact.

3) **Buspar (Buspirone):** This unique medication is a serotonin 1A partial agonist. It is well known that serotonin

plays a role in anxiety, which is why SNRIs and SSRIs (formerly known as antidepressants, though they go way beyond treating just depression, with multiple amazing "off-label" benefits) are first-line agents for anxiety disorders. Buspar seems to work better when added to another serotonergic agent and seems to be better for more generalized anxiety disorders rather than for more acute treatment of anxiety. I have prescribed it intermittently over the years, but I have not found it to be very effective for most of the patients that I have tried it on, though it has led to success for some. It tends to be more effective if the dose is increased to 30 mg twice a day instead of the "average" dose of 15 mg twice a day. I've not found it to be the best first- or second-line agent, but it is one to consider if there is still significant residual anxiety despite treatment with other potentially more effective medications.

4) **Dopaminergic agents:** I start thinking about this chemical more as related to anxiety and somatic disorders if I've already explored the other three more key neurochemicals and if anxiety symptoms still persist. Since anxiety and somatic disorders relate so closely to depressive disorders, it is not surprising that "atypical" medications in this class, which basically are dopamine and serotonin antagonists, may help, especially in more severe and treatment-resistant cases. In the majority of more difficult-to-resolve cases, there is related bipolar disorder, whether it is type 1, type 2, or bipolar spectrum disorder, which I will be discussing next.

Wellbutrin XL (the bupropion form I prescribe the most) is the other dopaminergic agent, which I use even more frequently as one of my primary augmenting agents for depression, though it is typically not useful for anxiety or somatic disorders. In fact, it can even increase anxiety. Therefore, with anxiety disorders, it plays more of a support role to add to other psychotropic medications that resolve anxiety, whether they be SNRIs, SSRIs, GABAergic medications of the "atypical" antipsychotic type, or whichever medication reduces anxiety but leads to lack of motivation and drive, sexual side effects, residual depression, difficulty losing weight, and other issues. It is a medication I often add in order to improve functioning and quality of life for many of my patients when a daily boost of dopamine is needed and appreciated.

Bipolar Disorders

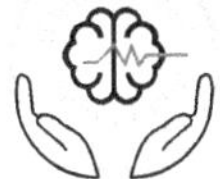

CHAPTER FOUR

Bipolar Disorders

Bipolar disorder, also known by the older term of manic-depressive illness, affects an individual's mood, behavior, and thinking. Depression and mania are often seen in an affective or mood spectrum. Affect is the external display of mood, whereas mood is an emotion felt internally. Mania and depression are "poles" apart. This has led to the terms "unipolar depression," for patients who experience a down or depressed mood, and "bipolar disorder," for patients who at different times experience the up or manic mood as well as the down or depressed mood. Depression and mania may even occur simultaneously, referred to as a "mixed" presentation. The symptoms vary as mood swings from the manic phase, characterized by feelings of elation, euphoria, extreme optimism, inflated self-esteem, delusional thinking, decreased need for sleep, a high tendency toward addictions, and many other signs, to the depressive phase, characterized by hopelessness, sadness, feelings of guilt, apathy, anhedonia, anxiety symptoms, suicidal ideation, and others. Many patients with bipolar disorder only experience the lower pole of depression, without experiencing the upper pole at all. I will be discussing this more in a bit.

I will review some definitions of terms important to understand in order to understand the full scope of bipolar disorder. I will then review DSM-5 criteria for some of the different types of bipolar disorder. I will discuss Bipolar I Disorder, Bipolar II Disorder, Cyclothymic Disorder, Bipolar Disorder Not Otherwise Specified (NOS), Bipolar Spectrum Disorder, and bipolar depression. I will then present a brief overview of bipolar disorder, followed by treatment recommendations.

Bipolar disorder is a fascinating subject that has an enormous impact on those who suffer with it. It is vastly under-recognized and undertreated. A frightful statistic I have heard is that it takes an average of three to four psychiatrists or other physicians seven to ten years to properly diagnose bipolar disorder. I'm not getting it; I wish I were. What a shame, and that is why it is so important to recognize that it involves various presentations, which are most often missed, and to learn how to recognize and treat it most completely and effectively.

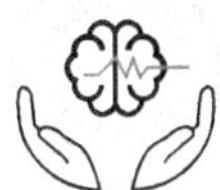

Mania

Acute mania is the hallmark symptom of bipolar disorder. What distinguishes Bipolar I Disorder from unipolar depression is the presence of at least one manic episode. The diagnostic criteria for a manic episode:

A. Persistent elevated, expansive, or irritable mood for at least one week (unless hospitalization is required).

B. At least three of the following symptoms are present during mood disturbance (four if mood is irritable):

- Inflated self-esteem or grandiosity.

- Decreased need for sleep.

- Increased talkativeness.

- Flight of ideas or racing thoughts.

- Easy distractibility.

- Increase in goal-directed activity or psychomotor agitation.

- Increase in risky behavior.

- Irritability and quickness to anger.

- Increased energy, activity, and euphoria.

- Loss of rationality, poor judgment, and unrealistic beliefs in one's abilities.

- Increased sexual urges and provocative behavior.

- Drug abuse, particularly alcohol, marijuana, benzodiazepines, and sleeping pills. Some are also drawn to stimulants, which can worsen the mania and lead to paranoia and irrational thinking, leading to significant instability and impairment.

C. Symptoms don't meet criteria for a mixed episode, which is when depression and mania occur simultaneously.

D. The level of illness is sufficient to cause social or occupational impairment, hospitalization, or psychotic features.

E. Symptoms are not due to a substance or medical condition.

Psychotic symptoms occur in at least 50% of manic episodes. In a delusional state, patients lose their perception of reality. For example, a person may believe they possess supernatural strength and ability, are extremely wealthy, or are publicly desired. Auditory hallucinations are common and can be dangerous, as these patients may also develop paranoia, which can lead to irrational behaviors, and may even present in the ER with florid grandiose psychosis with paranoid features, sometimes leading to violence if irritability is significant. Substance abuse can further disinhibit the person. So-called crimes of passion have been committed by patients harboring delusions of infidelity on the part of spouses or others, especially when under the influence of alcohol or another addictive substance.

Acute mania is a serious condition that needs to be recognized and treated quickly and correctly in order to stabilize the mood and the situation. Noncompliance is not unusual if the person feels euphoric and enjoys the state that his or her mind is in and does not want that to be disrupted. They may feel that medications will just bring them down and ruin a good thing. Since they often lack insight, they often do not understand that something is wrong and why it needs to be treated. When alcohol or other substances are introduced, the mind can become even more irrational, and the danger may then escalate. If we don't treat patients properly, then they will tend to treat themselves when it comes to acute mania.

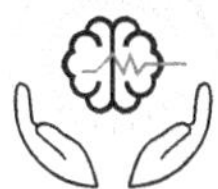

Hypomania

Hypomania refers to a mild to moderate presentation of mania. I refer to it as "mania lite," which is a "softer" presentation of mania. Hypomanic individuals may feel fantastic and even associate their symptoms with optimal functioning and enhanced productivity. It can be difficult to distinguish a hyperthymic personality who has a lot of energy and gets a lot done from hypomania. Friends and family members may notice the difference and warning signs, while the individual may deny there is anything wrong since they may lack insight. Hypomania is similar to mania; however, it is not serious enough to cause social or occupational impairment, hospitalization, or psychotic features. Hypomania also may be mistaken for anxiety, though with anxiety the individual typically knows there is something wrong.

Not distinguishing between anxiety and hypomania is probably one of the biggest sources of misdiagnosis between unipolar disorder and bipolar disorder. Without proper treatment of hypomania, this may lead to more severe mania, depression, mixed episodes, and mood instability in general. In addition to hypomania, the other symptom of depression may not be appreciated as the lower pole of bipolar disorder but rather considered as unipolar disorder. Doctors tend to focus too much on acute mania and not enough on hypomania and different types of depression as they relate to bipolar disorder. Most patients come in when they're depressed, not when they're hypomanic or manic. This is why a complete history is so important. Noncompliance with treatment is common, since these patients may enjoy the state of mind and not want to be brought down to a more "normal state." Patients don't tend to treat themselves in the correct preventative way unless they perceive that something is wrong that needs correcting

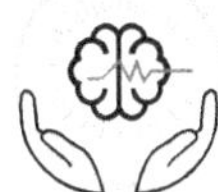

Mixed Episodes

This is when manic and depressive symptoms occur together. Symptoms of a mixed bipolar state often include agitation, restlessness, trouble sleeping, a significant change in appetite, psychosis, and suicidal thinking. A person may have a very sad and hopeless mood while at the same time feeling extremely energized and agitated. Mixed episodes are often severe and impair daily functioning in social interactions, occupational activity, and intimate relationships. The mixed episode can last from one week to several months and is generally followed by a severe depressive episode. Women are more prone to mixed episodes than men are. In teenagers, mixed episodes occur most frequently among those who have experienced major depression already, and for children, this may be the primary presentation of a mood disorder.

Momentary tearfulness and even depressed mood are commonly observed at the height of mania or during the transition from mania to depression, and these transient labile periods, which occur in most patients with Bipolar I Disorder, are different than actual mixed episodes. The latter, referred to as mixed mania or dysphoric mania, is characterized by dysphoric excited moods, irritability, anger, panic attacks, pressured speech, agitation, severe insomnia, grandiosity, hypersexuality, persecutory delusions and confusions, and suicidal ideation. This condition needs to be recognized and treated quickly, preferably with mood stabilizers initially for most cases, though antidepressants will likely follow at some point, which just depends on the history and presentation.

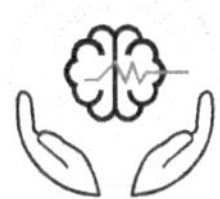

Rapid Cycling

When mania occurs at least four times per year, on average every few months, it is called rapid cycling. Patients with Bipolar I Disorder can also have rapid switches from mania to depression and back. Even though by definition this occurs at least four times a year, it can also occur much more frequently than that, as well as less frequently for some. This is a serious and dangerous condition, as are all the symptoms related to mania and mood instability. It's important to diagnose and treat this condition aggressively, usually leading with mood stabilizers and following with antidepressants, though it could be the other way around depending on the presentation and situation.

Now that we're familiar with the terminology, I will now review the other diagnostic criteria for the different bipolar disorders. I will then summarize my thoughts. As is the case with all of the mood disorders, including depression and anxiety, there is a lot of overlap between the different types of bipolar disorders as well as co-mingling with anxiety disorders, depressive disorders, ADD/ADHD, eating disorders, and other abnormal variations of mood and functioning. I will start with the most serious presentation of Bipolar I Disorder, followed by the lesser variations, though all of the variations are important to recognize in order to make the best diagnostic and treatment decisions.

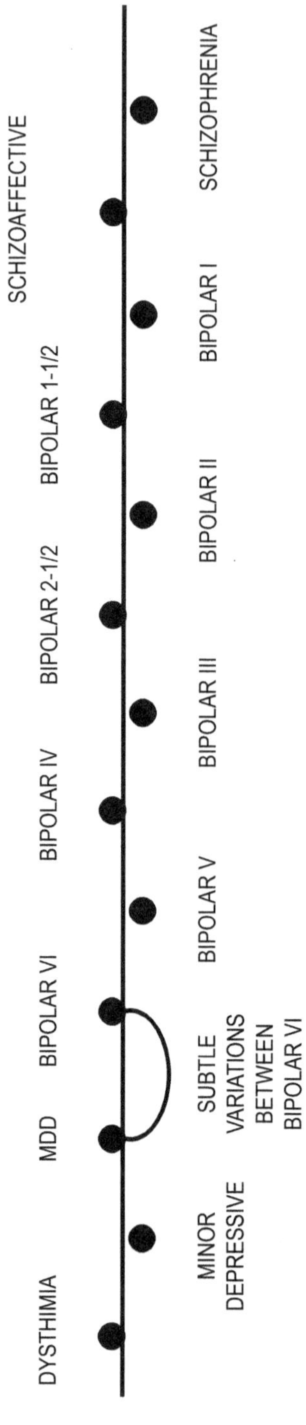
DYSTHIMIA
MINOR
DEPRESSIVE
MDD
BIPOLAR VI
BIPOLAR V
SUBTLE
VARIATIONS
BETWEEN
BIPOLAR VI
BIPOLAR IV
BIPOLAR III
BIPOLAR 2-1/2
BIPOLAR II
BIPOLAR 1-1/2
BIPOLAR I
SCHIZOAFFECTIVE
SCHIZOPHRENIA

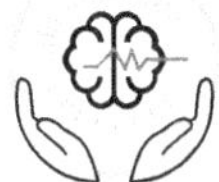

Bipolar I Disorder

Definition

A. Criteria have been met for at least one manic or mixed episode.

B. The symptoms cause social/occupational stress or impairment.

C. The symptoms are not better accounted for by schizoaffective disorder and are not superimposed on schizophrenia, schizophreniform disorder, delusional disorder, or psychotic disorder not otherwise specified.

Bipolar I is the most serious type of bipolar disorder with the highest risks. This disorder may be described as occurring on a continuum of severity ranging from mild forms of depression with brief mania to severe depression with rapid cycling mania. There is an enormous variation when it comes to bipolar disorders. Psychotic features may also accompany episodes of severe mania and depression. The aggressiveness of treatment depends on the presenting situation, by taking an excellent history regarding not only current symptoms but also the course of the illness from the beginning and along the way. The rockier the course, the more likely we are dealing with a bipolar disorder.

Discussion

I have seen estimates that approximately 1%, more or less, of the population has Bipolar I Disorder, which comprises about 10% of bipolar disorder. About 2% of the population has Bipolar II (Bipolar 2) Disorder, accounting for approximately 20% of bipolar disorder, which I will discuss next. About 70% of bipolar cases, more or less, are classified as Bipolar Disorder Not Otherwise Specified. Another term I really like and use a lot is "bipolar spectrum disorder." Bipolar III (Bipolar 3) through Bipolar VI (Bipolar 6), more or less, comprises the full range of subtle variations of bipolar disorder. That's estimated by many as about 10% of the population that has bipolar disorder, though I estimate that from the most subtle to the most severe. The key is proper recognition, since the more we recognize the subtleties, the higher that number will go.

Manic episodes are more common in men and outnumber the depressive episodes, while women have more depressive episodes than manic ones. In men depression may come out as irritability and anger more than in women, though this is difficult to generalize since it depends on the individual. There is a lot of variation in presentation within the bipolar spectrum. The more subtle variations (the "softer" presentations) are the ones that are missed the most by clinicians and by patients because they are so subtle and thus difficult to interpret. These are the ones that are most underdiagnosed and most undertreated, so it is so important for clinicians to recognize and appreciate the full range and impact of bipolar disorders. After we go through the other criteria, I will summarize my thoughts about bipolar disorder before I discuss my treatment strategies.

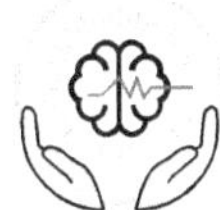

Bipolar II Disorder

A. Presence (or history) of one or more major depressive episodes.

B. Presence (or history) of at least one hypomanic episode.

C. There has never been a manic episode or a mixed episode.

D. The mood symptoms in Criteria A and B are not better accounted for by schizoaffective disorder, delusional disorder, or psychotic disorder not otherwise specified.

E. The symptoms cause clinically significant distress or impairment in social, occupational, or other important areas of functioning.

Specify current or most recent episode:

Hypomanic: If currently (or most recently) in a hypomanic episode.

Depressed: If currently (or most recently) in a major depressive episode.

Bipolar II Disorder is characterized by high episodes of euphoria and low episodes of depression. The depression could be classified as "hypodepression" or dysthymia or as the classic major depressive disorder. Hypomania differs from mania in two important respects. Hypomania can affect functioning and quality of life in all facets of life in an individual with Bipolar II Disorder. However, it is not as severe as manic episodes, which may require hospitalization in extreme cases or run-ins with the law. Hypomania does not involve psychosis and other severe irrational thinking. When the individual is hypomanic, he or she is more functional and still fairly rational, though not completely.

The current criteria specify that hypomania of four days is required to have the diagnosis. Currently the thinking is that two to three days may be enough to qualify, though in my opinion even one day is significant. As I said previously, the underdiagnosis of hypomania is one of the key reasons for the underdiagnosis of bipolar disorder and the overdiagnosis of unipolar disorder. Any kind of significant instability of mood is a tipoff that they fall within the bipolar spectrum.

Bipolar II, as well as all of the other variations, can have a major impact on quality of life. Hypomania, mood, and depressive episodes can influence daily functioning. Adaptation strategies and behavioral changes can help an individual to manage moods and remain balanced. Establishing the correct combination of medications and making sure that there are no significant side effects can have a significant impact on the person's quality of life.

Occupational functioning can be a significant problem for those who experience hypomania and depression, as is obviously the case with the even worse presentation of Bipolar I Disorder. They may have problems with concentration and with socializing with others at work. Employment rates may be lower as a result, since hypomania can lead to instability with work performance as well as working with others. The person may be stigmatized and may need to take more time off than the average person, which can potentially lead to the loss of a job. This condition can also lead to problems in relationships with friends as well as loved ones. Instability of mood can lead to instability of life in general. Proper treatment can provide that stability that is so desperately needed.

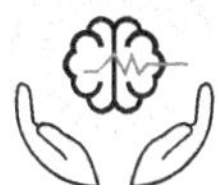

Schizoaffective Disorder

Before I discuss lesser variations of bipolar disorder, I want to briefly discuss schizoaffective disorder. I wasn't sure where to put this, since this is an even more serious condition than Bipolar I Disorder, but I wanted to start this section with the "classic" variation. I have referred to bipolar disorder as "schizophrenia lite," since they share certain features. The mania associated with Bipolar I Disorder can present with psychotic features, paranoia, delusional thinking, and even hallucinations. I will not be formally discussing schizophrenia in this book, but I wanted to list this variation between Bipolar I Disorder and schizophrenia since it is at the most extreme end of the full spectrum of bipolar disorder. I will first list the formal diagnostic criteria of schizoaffective disorder, followed by a brief discussion, before I then move on to the less extreme variations of the bipolar spectrum.

> A. An uninterrupted period of illness during which, at some time, there is either a major depressive episode, a manic episode, or a mixed episode con-

current with symptoms that meet Criterion A for schizophrenia. (These criteria are two or more characteristic symptoms of schizophrenia present for a significant portion of time during a one-month period, or less if successfully treated: delusions, hallucinations, disorganized speech, grossly disorganized or catatonic behavior, or negative symptoms, such as affective flattening.

B. During the same period of illness, there have been delusions or hallucinations for at least two weeks in the absence of prominent mood symptoms.

C. Symptoms that meet criteria for a mood episode are present for a substantial portion of the total duration of the active and residual periods of the illness.

D. The disturbance is not due to the direct physiological effects of a substance (e.g., a drug of abuse, a medication) or a general medical condition.

Specify type:

Bipolar type: If the disturbance includes a manic or mixed episode (or a manic or mixed episode and major depressive episodes).

Depressive type: If the disturbance only includes major depressive episodes.

This condition can be distinguished from bipolar I with psychotic mania by taking a thorough history and by following the course of the disease over time, as a higher degree may not be apparent initially. The prognosis of schizoaffective disorder is not quite as bad as schizophrenia but is worse than the prognosis for Bipolar I Disorder. I've seen this condition referred to as Bipolar 1/2 (Bipolar 0.5), which refers to a higher degree of mental illness than Bipolar I. This just goes to show that there is a continuum in the mental disease spectrum between psychotic disorders and mood disorders.

Schizophrenia is a chronic and unremitting illness, with often a poor prognosis and outcome and the decline in functioning over time, while bipolar disorder is a cyclical illness with often a better outcome and good restoration of function between episodes. Schizoaffective disorder falls somewhere in-between, and of course the outcome depends on the individual and the response to treatment, as well as how one does over time.

Now I'm going to resume the lesser forms of bipolar disorder as compared to schizoaffective disorder, bipolar I, and bipolar II. I will first list criteria for cyclothymic disorder, then bipolar disorder not otherwise specified, and then we will finish this section with a discussion of bipolar spectrum disorder.

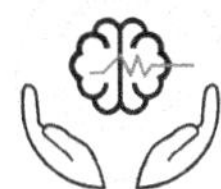

Cyclothymic Disorder

A. For at least 2 years, the presence of numerous periods with hypomanic symptoms and numerous periods with depressive symptoms that do not meet criteria for a major depressive episode. **Note:** In children and adolescents, the duration must be at least 1 year.

B. During the previously mentioned 2-year period (1 year in children and adolescents), the person has not been without the symptoms in Criterion A for more than 2 months at a time.

C. No major depressive episode, manic episode, or mixed episode has been present during the first 2 years of the disturbance. **Note:** After the initial 2 years (1 year in children and adolescents) of cyclothymic disorder, there may be superimposed manic or mixed episodes (in which case Bipolar I Disorder and cyclothymic disorder may be diagnosed) or major depressive episodes (in which case Bipolar II Disorder and cyclothymic disorder may be diagnosed).

D. The symptoms in Criterion A are not better accounted for by schizoaffective disorder and are not superimposed on schizophrenia, schizophreniform disorder, delusional disorder, or psychotic disorder not otherwise specified.

E. The symptoms are not due to the direct physiological effects of a substance (e.g., a drug of abuse or a medication) or a general medical condition (e.g., hypothyroidism).

F. The symptoms cause clinically significant distress or impairment in social, occupational, or other important areas of functioning.

This form of bipolar disorder often begins insidiously before 21 years of age and is characterized by frequent short cycles of milder depression, such as dysthymia or what I refer to as "hypo-depression" (depression lite) and hypomania (mania lite). The course of cyclothymia is either continuous or intermittent, with infrequent periods of euthymia (normal mood). The shifts of mood seen in this condition often occur with no precipitating reason. These patients may lead unstable lives by going in and out of relationships and may struggle at work and socially with friends and family. They may relocate frequently for a job or romantic relationship and then quickly lose interest and leave in frustration. They also often self-medicate with drugs and alcohol, which just exacerbates the situation. They tend to lead unstable lives in general.

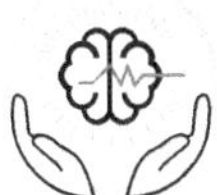

Bipolar Disorder Not Otherwise Specified

Bipolar disorder not otherwise specified (NOS) includes disorders with bipolar features that do not meet criteria for any specific type of bipolar disorder. Examples include the following:

1. Rapid alteration (over days) between manic symptoms and depressive symptoms that meet symptom threshold criteria but not minimal duration criteria for manic, hypomanic, or major depressive episodes.

2. Recurrent hypomanic episodes without intercurrent depressive symptoms.

3. A manic or mixed episode superimposed on delusional disorder, residual schizophrenia, or psychotic disorder not otherwise specified.

4. Hypomanic episodes, along with chronic depressive symptoms, that are too infrequent to qualify for a diagnosis of cyclothymic disorder.

5. Situations in which the clinician has indicated that a bipolar disorder is present but is unable to determine whether it is primary, due to a general medical condition, or substance-induced.

Bipolar disorder not otherwise specified (NOS) was in the DSM-IV, but they removed it from the DSM-5. I list it though because it is the closest to the newer term bipolar spectrum disorder, which I will discuss next. I traveled to a speaker training program to discuss the use of Seroquel (quetiapine) and Seroquel XR (quetiapine ER) while preparing us to lecture to other doctors about the product. At that time, there were three main categories for bipolar disorder: Bipolar I (about 10% of cases), Bipolar II (about 20%), and Bipolar NOS (about 70%). The high number of people in the NOS category—comprising roughly two-thirds to three-quarters of all cases—was striking both then and now. I asked the speaker at the time why we couldn't discuss Bipolar II or NOS, and I saw some doctors smiling and some chuckling. We all knew the reason was that the psychotropic medication we were discussing was formerly only indicated for treatment of Bipolar I Disorder. The speaker didn't want to discuss "off-label" indications or usage, since the FDA did not want me or other speakers to discuss "off-label" content, which is expressly prohibited. This is why so many doctors and other prescribers often don't understand the full value of these medications. They may not understand that "off-label" prescribing is the cutting edge in this field of medicine. This is why I am so passionate about speaking out and teaching others these vitally important topics.

However, since 90% of bipolar disorder is not Bipolar I, it is important for clinicians to understand the full spectrum of this disorder and how important it is to recognize the different variations and treat them appropriately. Thankfully we still have free speech in this country, though it is certainly threatened. I will speak out freely the best way I can to raise awareness about this important topic and the need for it to be discussed and then properly recognized and treated.

The DSM-5 has replaced Bipolar NOS by defining major depressive episodes with several sub-threshold conditions of bipolarity. For instance, allowing a duration of two to three days for hypomanic episodes, or fewer than four symptoms of hypomania during four days, or for cyclothymia allowing shorter manifestations (less than 24 months). Another important step is the recognition that dysthymia can co-occur with hypomania, which is considered a comorbid condition, or it could just be a variant of cyclothymic disorder. It's all so closely linked that it's difficult to separate these subtle variations.

If we are not free to discuss these variations openly due to FDA regulations, which I try to ignore, then bipolar disorder will continue to be the most underrecognized and undertreated disorder that I discuss, by far. It takes too many years and too many doctors in order to properly recognize, diagnose, and treat the many variations of bipolar disorder, which I firmly believe affects at least 10% of the population, and likely even more than half of patients with major depressive disorder and/or anxiety disorders have a coexisting variation of bipolar disorder.

The problem with the DSM-5 is that if we define the bipolar variations too narrowly, then the majority of the cases will be missed. Missing the difference between hypomania and high anxiety or subtle depression is one of the reasons for missing a large percentage of bipolar cases if we get too strict with our definitions and categorizations. We need to be able to step back and see the bigger picture and then do the right things for our patients based on the most complete evaluation, which leads to the best insight, knowledge, and judgment.

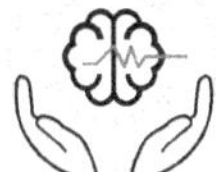

Bipolar Spectrum Disorder

This is not a formal disorder recognized in the DSM-5 but rather one that I made up. I like this term since it signifies that there is a spectrum when it comes to the multiple variations of bipolar disorder. This is a similar concept to the more newly defined Autistic Spectrum Disorder, which did make the DSM-5 and consists of variations between mild, moderate, and severe. That is exactly the same concept when it comes to the different variations of bipolar disorder. The most severe variations are severe Bipolar I Disorder and even worse Schizoaffective Disorder. Another term I like is "schizobipolar disorder." The moderate variations are milder Bipolar I, Bipolar II, and Cyclothymic Disorder (which I used to refer to as Bipolar III Disorder). Milder versions are also described by the current formal definitions of Bipolar III, IV, V, and VI, with more likely to come.

There is just so much individuality that it can be difficult to confine a clinical presentation of a person to a simple number. I have seen various definitions for different types and subtypes of bipolar disorder over the years, and I will list some of them but not all, in order to not be redundant. The take-home point here, though, is that there is so much similarity with subtle differences between the different variations within the bipolar spectrum. There is a richness and complexity to their symptoms and stories, and they are quite easily recognized if you know what to look for, and the answers are actually quite simple. For more information about bipolar disorder, see chapter 10, "The Ups and Downs of Bipolar Disorder," in the first book of my *Healing the Mind and Body* trilogy series. Let's now look at some of the subtypes that have informally been defined over the years:

Bipolar I: Depression and Mania

Bipolar 1 1/2: Depression with protracted hypomania

Bipolar II: Depression and Hypomania

Bipolar II 1/2 (2 1/2): Depression superimposed on cyclothymic temperament

Bipolar III: Cyclothymia is still what I refer to it as, but I've also seen Bipolar 3 referred to as antidepressant-caused hypomania.

Bipolar IIIa (3a): Depression and/or hypomania caused by substance use

Bipolar IV: Depression superimposed on a hyperthymic temperament

Bipolar V: Recurrent depression and dysphoric hypomania episodes or depression with mixed hypomania, euphoric, and/or dysphoric

Bipolar VI: Depression and bipolarity that
progress to a dementia-like disorder
like pseudo-dementia

As you can see, there is definite variation between the sub-groups along the bipolar spectrum. An important and interesting topic is when hypomania or mania is created by an antidepressant or illicit substance. My personal view is that if the upper pole is set off by a substance, that is a strong hint that there is an underlying smoldering predisposition toward at least bipolar spectrum disorder as the true underlying disorder. That is essentially what leads to self-medicating or being medicated improperly by a clinician who is giving an antidepressant when a mood stabilizer is actually the better choice, or at least an augmenting choice. The good thing is that this recognition leads to a change of the diagnosis and to improvement in the treatment, hopefully.

The other lower variants of bipolar disorder shared features of instability of mood in general, antidepressant-induced mood cycling, substance-induced mood cycling, or anyone with excessive mood swings, which leads to instability in life. Some patients only have mania or hypomania without the onset of depression. They may not see the need for formal treatment if they are only experiencing the upper pole of mood, and if they are on a roll, they don't want it to stop. They may be successful and not see any need to treat it, since they don't want anything to bring them down. They tend to self-medicate with addictive substances, especially if they are not treated adequately. They may never seek treatment if they believe their lives are going well and that there is no need for any type of change. The problem is, though, that the high of mania or hypomania does not last, and then the risk is the crash into depression. The higher the high often results in the lower of the low afterwards.

This may happen during the adolescent years, but it is even more likely during midlife, when hormonal imbalances coexist with underlying genetic factors and situational stressors during the 40s and 50s. I often see, though, that the risk actually increases in women and also men in the mid- to late 30s, which I classify as pre-perimenopausal in women. That time of life is significant when it comes to the onset or worsening of an underlying problem. I refer to men in their 40s to 50s as having male menopause, which I jokingly refer to as "Manopause" or "midlife crisis." This is when testosterone may be declining, while for women mood may have to do with the slow decrease of estrogen and other hormones. The hormones in general of both sexes lead to change most significantly during the 40s and 50s, and prior to that would be puberty, the most significant initial hormone imbalance, which can be a rocky time for some, along with PMDD and postpartum for some women. That's why these times of life, in my experience, are the most common times of onset and worsening of conditions related to neurochemical imbalances.

Bipolar IV (Bipolar 4) is interesting, since it may be difficult to tell the difference between someone with a hyperthymic temperament and someone who has hypomanic or manic tendencies. Patients with hyperthymia are often successful, sunny, optimistic, high-output people, and some stay that way without crossing the line. However, some of them at some point split off into one direction or the other, such as depression, hypomania, mania, or any other variants of the disorder.

Is a hyperactive or irritable and moody teenager normal or abnormal? It really depends on if they are really just not themselves and if it is affecting the person's functioning. If the adolescent is turning toward illicit drugs, is hanging out with the wrong crowd, is engaging in high-risk activities, is suffering academically, or has suicidal ideation, then these are all signs that an urgent evaluation and treatment are advisable.

Therapy as well as medications can both be helpful during these formative years. Whether at this stage, during midlife, or whenever it occurs, if the "up" and hypercharged mood remain within a rational range, it may be the person's normal. However, if it crosses into anger, irritability, irrational mania, or more rational hypomania, intervention with a mood stabilizer is advisable in order to start tuning the person down. Some have a crossover in-between Bipolar I and II, shifting from low-grade mania to hypomania to depression. The absence of true mania is what distinguishes II from I.

Bipolar V (Bipolar 5) is not really any different than the other disorders along the bipolar spectrum. Having depression and mixed hypomania just sounds like typical bipolar spectrum stuff to me. Depression and hypomania often seem to come together to cause disruption at both poles. Hypomania in particular can be very difficult to discern if you're not looking for it. It can be episodic or chronic and may not affect the mood negatively at all if you're lucky. It can also, though more commonly, lead to irritability and anger. Younger kids tend to present with irritability, anger, and destructiveness instead of the euphoric mania, while adults tend toward both mania and irritability, sometimes at the same time. Shortening the hypomanic phase to two to three days instead of four days may help one to recognize that the amount of time really doesn't matter. Even one day or less of symptoms is enough to warrant treatment of the suffering individual. What matters most is that there is a problem to fix, and we have more than adequate tools to work with in order to make that happen.

In these situations and others, I consider bipolar spectrum disorder the most likely diagnosis until proven otherwise. Most people with this condition spend more time in depression than they do in hypomania or mania, especially women. If the patient presents with depression, it's imperative to take a detailed history of previous changes in mood, starting at the beginning. Talking to friends and loved ones of the patient is often critical, because they more easily see what the patient doesn't see as significant. If there is a history of instability of life in the past and/or current instability, then the treatment plan can completely change lives for the better, thus leading to better results and happier patients.

Bipolar VI (Bipolar 6) can also be another subtle presentation. Some patients who experience dementia actually have pseudo-dementia, which can be the onset symptoms of a mood disorder. Some patients may have coexisting dementia and a mood disorder, both requiring treatment. Certain mental health issues get worse with age and especially with dementia, so proper recognition and treatment are vital. Depending on the situation, we need to be aware of whether we are prescribing antidepressants, mood stabilizers, or both. In these cases, a combination of both classes of medications is the ideal treatment and the strategy that most likely leads to full remission.

I'm sure that in the future we will be coming up with other numbers and letters in order to be able to describe all of the different variations and subtle hints that describe different types and subtypes of this disorder. The most important takeaway point here is that not all patients with depression have major depressive disorder. If the history and treatment course do not go as planned, then we need to reconsider the diagnosis and rethink the treatment plan. Bipolar spectrum disorder encompasses the multiple various presentations, from subtle to more obvious, from mild to moderate to severe. Since symptomatic patients with bipolar disorder spend much more of their time in the depressed state rather than the manic, hypomanic, or mixed state, that's why so many depressed patients in the past and currently are treated for unipolar disorder, leading to poor or incomplete response to treatment. Antidepressant monotherapy does not work well for these patients.

An antidepressant may give very quick positive results, which then "poop out," may worsen the condition, or may improve the condition only incompletely, without achieving full remission. If the response to an antidepressant is "too good too quickly," this can be a warning sign of potential mania, instability, and even suicidal risk. The addition of a mood stabilizer, or even a couple together with one or two antidepressants, should be the typical treatment strategy. We'll discuss this in more detail in a bit. In some patients monotherapy with a mood stabilizer is appropriate. It just depends on the individual.

Antidepressant therapy can worsen mood cycling, mixed states, and conversion to hypomania and mania. It may even increase suicidal thinking, so this needs to be screened for and closely monitored. Thus, it is important to recognize whether the depressed patient has a bipolar spectrum disorder or a unipolar major depression. The reality is that patients with either unipolar or bipolar depression often have currently identical symptoms, which is why taking a detailed history, including the past mood symptoms and patterns, tried and failed medications, a detailed family history, and the difference of previous symptoms as compared to the current ones, is important.

Regarding past history, I look for instability of life and hints of cyclical changes over time, along with responses to previous treatments such as antidepressants. The family history is more "loaded" for bipolar patients than for unipolar patients. There is also a higher addiction rate for bipolar patients as compared to unipolar patients, though this is a big problem for both. A past family history of suicide also tends toward the possibility of bipolarity. If one has a history of mood disorders on both sides of the family, then the like-lihood is that your mood disorder will be worse. It's difficult to know for many relatives if they had a mood disorder or not, but signs of instability in life are a hint that there was an underlying problem.

Another important factor is to get a history from a friend or loved one that knows the person very well and can thus give important and impactful information that the patient may not share, since that person may not see it as a problem and think it's just normal or maybe be in denial. They also may be embarrassed about sharing certain information. Patients tend to under-report their manic and hypomanic symptoms, and they may have poor insight and occasionally irrational thinking and behaviors that may not be obvious during the interview. They tend to focus on their depression, anxiety, and stress symptoms, as well as somatic symptoms. Someone who knows the patient can give excellent insight into what that person's "normal" is really like, which is so helpful because they know that person way better than I do. When these patients are "just not themselves," we need to find out why and get them back to normal as quickly and safely as we can.

Another vital factor pertaining to unipolar and bipolar disorder is the hormonal status of the patient. The most common time of onset of bipolar disorder is mid- to late adolescence, such as 15 to 19 years, though bipolar disorder can be seen in young to older children, people in middle age, and older adults. Women tend to have more depressive episodes and mixed episodes, while men tend more toward manic episodes, though both sexes experience both. Women have more times of hormonal changes than men do, which is why depression and bipolar disorder are more common in women; however, men still get their fair share. The peak times are puberty, premenstrual, postpartum, pre- and perimenopausal, menopausal, and postmenopausal. In men and women, puberty/teenage years and midlife are the two most common times of onset and worsening. As I said, for men during the 40s and 50s, I call the hormonal change "manopause" or "midlife crisis."

Women also tend to seek out help and be more open to treatment than men are. Women tend to be better listeners and communicators, and they understand better that something is wrong in their bodies that needs attention. Men are more likely not to recognize that they have a problem, and they are less likely to seek and follow through with treatment. These are, of course, generalizations, since many women also are averse to being "labeled" and treated when they really should be.

Another factor that may play a role in unipolar and bipolar disorders is an environmental factor, such as weather, humidity, and other factors. For example, for people who live in climates that are rainier and colder, the incidence of depression is higher than if one were living in a sunny and warm environment. Seasonal Affective Disorder (SAD) is most common during the holiday season, especially when it gets dark earlier and the days are shorter. The holidays also bring back memories of the past with family and friends. Sometimes these memories are not so good, and the remembrances of good and bad times are more vivid and real during the holidays between Halloween and New Year's. Whether the memories are good or bad, the feelings about them seem to intensify during the last couple months of the year.

However, some people cycle at different times of the year and can tend to get more manic during the spring to summer and more depressed the latter part of the year, though it is difficult to simplify it in this way since everyone's experience is different. These are just generalizations, though, and not true for all people.

Bipolar patients who rapid cycle have at least four cyclical episodes throughout the year, though some may cycle more frequently than that or less frequently than that. Cycling of mood is a sure tipoff that we are dealing with bipolar disorder, and the details of the cycles are very important in order to understand the full extent of the mood disorder. There are other environmental factors also besides just the amount of sunlight, though not all of the contributors are well understood at this point. It's encouraging, though, that we are learning more and more at such a rapid rate. It is certainly exciting to be involved in learning and teaching the methods that I have developed over time.

There are so many symptoms that may suggest bipolar spectrum disorder, which include excessive drowsiness, overeating, overdrinking or abusing drugs, motor retardation, mood lability, anger, irritability, or suicidal ideation, as well as others. There are hints that the depression may be in actuality Bipolar Spectrum Disorder, which include the course of the untreated illness prior to the current symptoms, the early age of onset, the degree of family history, the high frequency of depressive episodes, a high proportion of the time spent ill, the intensity and duration of the symptoms, paranoia, fear, rage, intense anger, panic attacks, phobias, and other obvious or subtle factors. The term "multipolar" disorder may be more appropriate for some of these patients.

The response to antidepressants gives crucial information in order to figure out the best treatment, which we can figure out due to past failures. Bipolar depression is more likely if there are multiple antidepressant failures, rapid recovery that isn't sustained by either crashing or "pooping out," or activating side effects such as jitteriness, nervousness, abnormal body movements, insomnia, loss of appetite, and anxiety. Another hint is the actual worsening of mood with an antidepressant. Another hint is if the person gets too well too quickly, which, as I just said, can lead to instability and increased risk. The point is to be vigilant to the possibility that what may at first look like a unipolar disorder may actually be along the spectrum of bipolar disorder instead. The different treatment approaches I will discuss later depend on the presentation and history. We then find out more as we go along and see how treatment goes, paying attention to the benefits as well as the side effects, while attempting to increase the former and decrease the latter.

Bipolar spectrum disorder is so important to recognize since it is so common, and the usual presentation of bipolar disorder is not Bipolar I or even Bipolar II, but rather somewhere else along the spectrum. They may present with "softer" symptoms than are seen with more severe variations of bipolar disorder. "Soft" bipolar disorder may present with a variety of symptoms such as depression, anxiety, somatic symptoms that are more erratic and change over time, and other symptoms that are not formally defined in the DSM-5. The hypomania is often more dysphoric than euphoric, and it is important to recognize that symptoms of depression are much more common than symptoms of hypomania and mania, though it is most common to have a mixture that presents in many unique ways.

As I already mentioned, hypomania can be either dysphoric or euphoric. Hypomania in patients with soft bipolar disorders can be either, but is usually dysphoric. Dysphoric hypomania is characterized by irritability, impulsiveness, and poor judgment, while euphoric hypomania can often be pleasant for the individual, causing them to have a temporary boost in productivity and positive emotions. Dysphoric symptoms can be quite damaging to relationships and the work environment and can be accompanied by a sense of desperation. Hypomania can often alternate with depression, making the mood of the individual highly unstable at certain times. The most common form of hypomania, namely dysphoric hypomania, can often be identified due to the bouts of paranoia, rage, and other emotions that the individual often experiences. Some individuals experience simultaneous hypomania and depression, which is known as mixed bipolar disorder. Some people have rapid cycles, and some people have slow cycles. The rate and intensity of the cycles depend on the presentation of the individual at hand.

Many bipolar spectrum patients have been previously prescribed anxiolytic medications and/or antidepressants by their family physician or their psychiatrist. They often don't have the desired response to these drugs, some only experiencing partial relief, some worsening, and some regressing into more intense episodes of depression, anxiety, hypomania, or mania. Some of these patients take high doses of benzodiazepines or other potentially addictive substances. This approach may or may not work, though in reality it is not the best and healthiest treatment for that individual. It's better to prevent and resolve the problem rather than to just cover it up by "Band-Aiding" it. Benzodiazepines are still useful, but better at lower doses and only as needed rather than regularly. *The more symptomatic medications the patient takes, the more likely they fall within the bipolar spectrum.*

Proper subtyping of bipolar spectrum disorder should be identified, accepted, and used by all clinicians who treat mood disorders, whether they be primary care practitioners (including family physicians, internists, pediatricians, PAs, and NPs), psychiatrists, or other specialists. We must go outside of the DSM-5 box in order to recognize all the fascinating varieties of presentations and learn how to treat them in the most complete way.

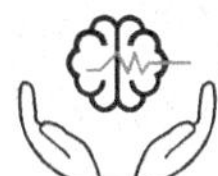

Comorbid Condition

There are a lot of comorbid conditions regarding bipolar disorder (as well as unipolar disorder) that I will review.

Over half of individuals with bipolar disorders are also living with other psychiatric and medical conditions. Comorbidity is the rule rather than the exception. This can make diagnosis and proper treatment more challenging, but I like a challenge. I will list the conditions that can impact the diagnosis and treatment of the bipolar disorders, as well as unipolar depression and anxiety disorders for that matter.

1) **Thyroid conditions:** Both hypothyroidism and hyperthyroidism can complicate the diagnosis and treatment of bipolar disorders. Since the symptoms associated with hyperthyroidism can emulate those of hypomania or even mania more rarely. This can both make bipolar disorder difficult to diagnose and make the symptoms more pronounced. On the other hand, hypothyroidism can often resemble the symptoms of depression, such as fatigue, apathy, lack of motivation, and other depressive symptoms.

This could be the reason why antidepressants are not always successful and may just cause side effects or even worsen the underlying condition. Another complicating factor is that lithium carbonate use may lead to hypothyroidism in some.

Subclinical hypothyroidism has been linked to the development of rapid cycling and mixed bipolar disorders, so there is a lot of interplay between thyroid and mood that we may not even completely understand. Since thyroid function is part of most screening panels, this is easy enough to diagnose and treat. Optimal treatment of thyroid conditions can certainly improve mood, so it is important to attend to this if it is an issue. If both the thyroid and mood disorder are not treated adequately at the same time, then the individual is unlikely to ever achieve full remission.

2) **Substance Abuse:** Alcohol and drug abuse are both common when it comes to bipolar disorder, even more so than with unipolar disorder, where the risk is still too high. In my estimation well more than half of patients with a bipolar spectrum disorder will struggle with significant substance abuse at some point in their lifetimes, if not at several points. This can be a significant issue, since addictive and intoxicating substances can worsen symptoms of bipolar disorder. These patients tend to "self-medicate" if we do not medicate them correctly in a preventative and curative way. Patients who are depressed may abuse not only alcohol but also stimulants, legal or illegal opiates, marijuana, hallucinogens, "party" drugs, and other substances that at least temporarily improve mood.

There are many self-medicating choices available, more and more over time. People who are anxious or manic may tend toward alcohol, marijuana, benzodiazepines, one of the opiates, and other types of relaxants. Nicotine and caffeine can also be abused when one is self-medicating, since both of them are so easily available. Even patients who partake of other drugs and alcohol have a difficult time beating cigarettes, since nicotine is one of the most addictive substances known to mankind. Caffeine is the most used legal substance, which can be overdone by some and can thus have an addictive component, whether it's coffee, tea, or "power drinks" and energy supplements, though most people keep caffeine intake to a more moderate and nonaddictive level. Those who abuse it may be more prone to anxiety, irritability, anger, and an overall imbalanced mood.

Drugs and alcohol can temporarily improve short-term anxiety and fatigue but cannot cause bipolar disorder when one does not have the underlying propensity toward it. It can, however, exacerbate it.

These patients often require a dual diagnosis evaluation and individualized treatment plan. Dual diagnosis means treating both the addiction and the underlying mood disorder at the same time. In my opinion this is almost always the case in addiction. There is usually some type of mood disorder, whether subtle or more obvious, that fuels the addiction. Bipolar disorder in particular definitely makes one more prone to have both mood and addiction issues at the same time. It is important to treat both adequately in order to achieve and maintain full remission.

Some experts recommend at least 30 days of optimal treatment of the addictions before psychotropic medications are introduced. I think that is too strict, though, since I tend to treat the bipolar disorder as soon as possible, even if the addictions are not fully resolved. I believe that optimal treatment of the neurochemical imbalances involved increases the chance of achieving and maintaining sobriety from illicit drugs and alcohol.

3) **Hypogonadism/low testosterone:** This is more common in middle-aged to older men, though it rarely happens also at a younger age. If a man presents with symptoms of low energy, low motivation and drive, depression, lack of or lowered sex drive, or other potential symptoms, then his testosterone level should be checked. If the testosterone level is low, then a testosterone supplement can boost mood, energy, motivation, sex drive, and sexual functioning. If the testosterone level is too high, such as in someone taking an illicit steroid, or if testosterone supplementation is really not needed but can easily be acquired on the street or from a shady operation where they can get way too much of the supplement, which includes topical forms but more likely high doses of injectables, then this can lead to mania or hypomania symptoms, increased anxiety and moodiness, as well as anger, irritability, and overall instability of mood. This is where the term "roid rage" comes from, since those who use a testosterone supplement when not needed are like taking a steroid in a way that is not therapeutic but rather abusive.

Even women who have low testosterone can see a negative effect on mood and energy, and testosterone replacement in their case may help their mood, energy, and sex drive, whereas if it is not needed, it may create more irritability and an imbalance of mood. Women also see a decrease in mood when estrogen is low, which is one reason why women experience depressive symptoms more than men do.

Supplementing hormones to men or women who need them can have a symbiotic effect with antidepressants and mood stabilizers in order to achieve the best and most complete results by treating all measurable aspects related to mood. Since hormonal imbalances are the second most important etiology of mood disorders, second to genetic predisposition, attention toward balancing hormones properly is a very important factor to address.

4) **ADD/ADHD** is typically associated with children who struggle to pay proper attention at school; however, it should be noted the symptoms also often happen when one grows up. It can affect work as well as communication skills, with the most important one being the ability to listen. This condition can negatively affect relationships also. The symptoms of this condition are poor focus and concentration due to easy distractibility, impulsivity, restlessness, hyperactivity, inattention. These symptoms are similar in certain aspects to those who suffer with bipolar disorder. However, bipolar symptoms are rarely constant, while one lives with ADHD symptoms most of the time in one form or another. It is important to

understand the difference, since the treatments for ADHD may worsen bipolar disorder, though in some it improves the situation. The treatment of bipolar disorder may worsen the ADHD symptoms in some, which necessitates the optimal treatment of both. If they exist together at the same time, then it is important that both disorders be treated optimally so that the best overall results are achieved. Treating both together is a bit trickier but well worth the results seen when it is done correctly.

5) **Personality Disorders:** Patients with Borderline Personality Disorder (BPD), a classic variant, often have varied symptoms that are included in the other personality disorders, such as histrionic and narcissistic traits; thus, they are on the borderline between different personality types, causing a combination of different aspects of personalities that present in unique ways. This disorder can cause significant problems functioning in life. Personality disorders overall in general are among the most difficult to treat when it comes to mental health, but there are others not far behind, such as eating disorders, severe OCD, addiction, and more severe bipolar variations. This personality type can make daily life difficult due to instability of mood and the overall presentation.

These individuals present in a more dramatic fashion medically, since their personality is often dramatic at the same time, leading to instability in life with regard to work, home, and play.

These patients are also prone to being very sensitive to criticism and have a fear of abandonment since other people really don't want to be around them when they act this way. People refer to them as "walking on eggshells" around them since they can be very annoying and exasperating to be around. They then become more desperate to hang on to anything that they can, leading to frustration that others are not willing to put up with, which is most people. This creates even more of a desperation in the person, trying desperately to hold on to whatever they need from a relationship. They often put too much pressure on loved ones and often have unrealistic demands of their families and friends. They tend to be a bit narcissistic and self-destructive, and suicidal ideation is not uncommon in this very unstable group of people.

The most important point that I want to emphasize here is the interplay between personality disorders and bipolar disorders. It's difficult, though, to separate these disorders that are so closely intertwined. The good news that I have discovered with these patients is that if we treat the underlying mood disorder correctly, then the more extreme features of the personality of the person can tend to mellow out a bit. Psychotropic medications may take away the "rough edges" of the personality and put the person more in control, since the psychotropic medications are preventative by actually correcting the core problem of neurochemical imbalances. Once these are corrected, then the person becomes more in control of his or her thoughts, emotions, and actions.

Psychotherapy of the right type can be helpful with BPD. Especially dialectical behavioral therapy (DBT), along with the right medication, can help to mellow out the personality a bit without actually changing the personality. The problem, though, is that many BPD patients do not recognize that they have a problem, which other people can quite easily recognize. They believe that that's just the way they are and that it is not a problem for them. They may believe that everybody else is the problem. They may not take ownership of their role in situations. The problem then falls on others who have to deal with the burden of being around them. They can be obnoxious, annoying, abrasive, obsessive, and hateful at times, and typically you don't want to be around the person once you get to know her or him. Dreading spending time with that person is a sure tipoff that BPD may be a significant issue that we need to consider and explore.

Psychotherapy, especially DBT (Dialectical Behavioral Therapy), can help these patients if they are willing to follow through with directions. If the personality and mood can work together, this makes for a much more functional life for these individuals. If the person is not as annoying and abrasive and is easier to be around, this hints that successful treatment was applied. Successful treatment usually means psychotherapy along with adequate medical treatment, which usually includes one or more antidepressants with one or more mood stabilizers, creating the ideal combination for that individual.

BPD is not the only personality disorder that is closely connected to all variants of bipolar disorder, since comorbidity is the rule rather than the exception. The different personality types include histrionic traits, narcissistic traits, paranoia, irrational thinking, hypochondria, phobias, passive aggressiveness, antisocial characteristics, and other variants of one's personality. When both the personality disorder and whichever type of bipolar disorder are both treated in an ideal fashion, then the results can be quite good. They can be difficult to treat, though, since they tend to be self-destructive, manipulative, and unwilling to see that they have a problem and voluntarily and actively seek treatment.

Substance abuse is quite common in this population, and both psychological and pharmacological therapies are very helpful, especially when combined properly. While part of them may understand that treatment is beneficial, they still may fight it and put up barriers to treatment rather than being more proactive in preventing the problem rather than needing to treat it after the fact.

Bipolar disorder and personality disorders are quite common in those who are incarcerated. Jails and prisons are the new psychiatric wards since they deinstitutionalized people with severe mental health issues decades ago. This can lead to homelessness and living in other unhealthy situations. Poor mental health also leads to an increased risk of risky behaviors, such as crime and drug abuse, which go hand-in-hand. One problem, though, is that prisoners usually get improper and inadequate medical treatment for their mental illnesses, even more than the general population. It's always better to prevent problems than to deal with them after the fact when the damage is already done. If we treat the underlying neurochemical imbalances that lead to mood disorders and contribute to personality disorders, then the substance abuse rate would go down, the crime rate would go down, and society would be more at peace.

Treatment of mood disorders definitely drives down the addiction rate and the crime rate and holds the best chance of leading a healthy life in sobriety and otherwise at peace. Proper treatment of neurochemical imbalances and addictions could most definitely reduce the prison population, transferring nonviolent addicts to drug rehabilitation rather than behind bars. Many of our prisoners would be better served by proper psychiatric and addiction care, which means treating the underlying problems that lead to these behaviors in the first place.

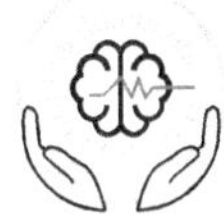

Summary

Bipolar disorder in all its various forms is, in my estimation, the most underappreciated, underrecognized, underdiagnosed, and undertreated medical problem that we know of. I don't think it is even close. The most common misdiagnoses are unipolar depressive or anxiety disorder instead of a bipolar spectrum disorder. The results of the treatment will signify whether the treatment works or not or if we were right after the fact. If the treatment gives incomplete results, makes the person feel worse, or does nothing, then this leads to frustration and potential noncompliance. The treatments are all very quick and easy to assess, which is a good aspect when it comes to these disorders. The switch to or the addition of a mood stabilizer is usually what makes the biggest difference. I will discuss medications next, but the mood stabilizers consist of a few groups of medications that we will discuss.

The depressive disorders are also varied in their presentations, so we need to take note of every detail and every piece of relevant information. It is vitally important for the clinician to pay close attention to all the details and clues in the patient's history and presentation and to understand the individuality of the patient and the specific needs and desires in order to achieve whichever combination of treatments to go on to provide the best results possible.

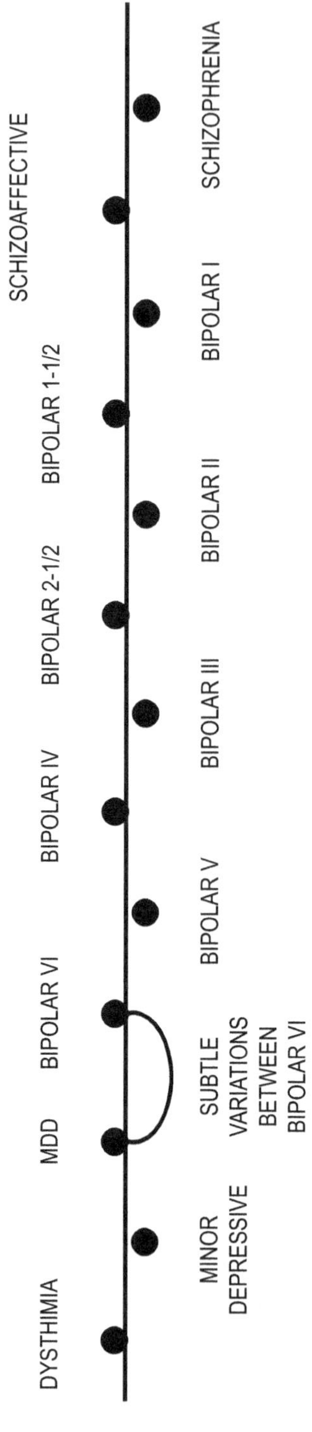

DYSTHIMIA
MDD
BIPOLAR VI
BIPOLAR IV
BIPOLAR 2-1/2
BIPOLAR 1-1/2
SCHIZOAFFECTIVE
MINOR
DEPRESSIVE
SUBTLE
VARIATIONS
BETWEEN
BIPOLAR VI
BIPOLAR V
BIPOLAR III
BIPOLAR II
BIPOLAR I
SCHIZOPHRENIA

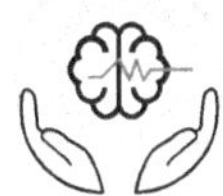

Starting Treatment

I have discovered that the best results are often a combination of more than one antidepressant and more than one mood stabilizer at the same time, leading to sometimes two but more often three to four or more medications together, as compared to sometimes one but usually two to three medications at once for unipolar disorder. There is so much interaction and detail that relates to each person that we treat, so we need to make sure to be in tune with all of the aspects that the patient needs at the same time. Clinicians who treat these disorders, whether physicians, PAs, or NPs, need to really get to know the details of each patient regarding his or her detailed history in order to best understand that patient in order to pick the most optimal treatment regimen in the right order. The natural inclination for most clinicians is to treat first-line with antidepressants.

This antidepressant-first approach is often appropriate for many but not for all. That is the case with many of them. If the problems are not treated adequately or just partially treated, then the person never really gets completely better. Treating everything needed at the same time is really the only way to reach our treatment goals, though this may not be easy to achieve unless it is done correctly. The more aggressive the treatment, the better, as long as the treatment course is safe and effective, which is what happens when the proper decisions are made.

My strategy is to make my best educated guess as to the first medication to try, and if it does not give the desired results or side effects are problematic, I will switch to another agent, and I will keep doing so until the best medication is optimally titrated before I add an augmenting agent. I don't like to do two things at once since it can then be confusing in regard to what is doing what. I titrate and augment aggressively since decisions are able to be made quickly with psychotropic medications. A common myth is that it takes psychotropic medications four to six to eight weeks to work, but that is simply not the case. Except for Lamictal (lamotrigine), most medications give results within the first week, definitely within the second week. The rational trial-and-error approach is the best scientific method to achieve the rational polypharmaceutical optimization.

There are a lot of people with some variation of bipolar disorder who are in desperate need of help that they are not getting. The better we get at recognizing the subtle variations and symptoms that relate to the mood and body, the more we realize that often several neurochemicals are involved at the same time, leading to a variety of presentations regarding the person's body, mind, and mood that come together. Treating the mind and body at the same time is crucial. The special needs of each individual are what really matter in the end, so whichever treatment approach it takes to achieve the ideal goals is worth the time it takes to achieve it. When the body and mind are both working together, there is no stopping that person from achieving true happiness.

Treatment of bipolar disorders involves patience with our patients. It takes a recognition that there are various reasons why the person is in your office needing help. The better we can diagnose properly and then treat them correctly at the same time, the better we can help them. The rational trial-and-error approach is the rule and not the exception when it comes to psychopharmacology. The rule is that the person has more than one neurochemical out of balance, and thus it takes more than one medication in order to fill the need. This requires the rational polypharmaceutical approach, which is the only way that we can really get to the answers that we seek. We make an educated guess as to what to try first, since we need to start somewhere. Once we see the initial reaction and the side effect profile, we can then decide which course to follow. This often takes follow-up visits in order to achieve the best results, which I'm usually able to achieve within two to three visits. If it takes three to six visits or more to get the patient to full remission, this means that this person is more difficult to treat, which increases the odds that we are dealing with some variation of bipolar disorder.

If the right antidepressant is not chosen quickly, then this delays the process. If it does not achieve positive results quickly without significant side effects, then this is a hint that we may not be dealing with unipolar disorder, though this also may mean that the wrong antidepressant was chosen and that we need to explore a different class of antidepressant. The likelihood when it comes to bipolar disorder is that at least one antidepressant will be needed since depression is such a large part of the disorder.

The problem is that the effects either don't last or are incomplete, and the obvious answer is that one or more mood stabilizers with one or more antidepressants will be needed in order to achieve the optimal result of complete mood stabilization. Those with addictive disorders coexisting with other mood disorders, especially bipolar disorder, are even more challenging to treat, but I like a challenge, and I love seeing the results when it is done just right. This can only be done, though, if we listen intently to our patients in order to make sure we do for them exactly what is needed.

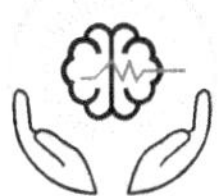

Treatment of Bipolar Disorders

Before starting treatment, it is imperative to get a detailed history, including a past history of mood disorders, a history of mood cycling or any evidence of instability of mood, a history of all of the psychotropic medications, including detailed descriptions of the benefits and side effects seen, a detailed family history, all current and past symptomatology, a history of past and current substance abuse, pertinent lab work, and other diagnostic studies. It also certainly helps to get information from family and close friends, who may notice things that the patient does not realize about him- or herself. The more detailed and complete the history, the better the diagnosis and treatment strategy.

1) Should we start with an antidepressant or a mood stabilizer? The answer to that question really depends on the history obtained and the current status of the patient as well as the recent past. Most patients present with symptoms of depression rather than hypomania or mania, and if that is the case, it is reasonable to start with an antidepressant. If the patient is rather at the upper pole, then starting

with a mood stabilizer is advisable. If the patient is in a mixed state with both the lower and upper poles at the same time, then a mood stabilizer is the safer bet. If the patient is unstable, switching back and forth in a rapid cycling fashion, then definitely a mood stabilizer would be the logical choice.

It may take more than one mood stabilizer in order to get the patient in a safer and more stable place. Choosing the right agent and learning to combine antidepressants and mood stabilizers is the art and science in this specialty of medicine. If an antidepressant is chosen and resolves the depression but pushes the patient into a hypomanic or manic state, we can choose to stop the antidepressant or continue it and quickly add a mood stabilizer. We need to be most careful if the patient has Bipolar I Disorder, whereas lesser variations are less likely to lead to significant instability. If the person is not unstable (meaning not in a high manic state with paranoia, irrational thinking, and/or suicidal ideation), then it is reasonable to continue the antidepressant and then augment. Antidepressants can tend to work quite quickly in bipolar patients, so we need to work quickly in order to make sure that both poles are stabilized.

On the other hand, if a mood stabilizer is chosen first, once the mania or hypomania is resolved, the patient may be left in a depressive state that needs attention. In that case I then add an antidepressant to try to pull the patient out of that state. Our patients need to know that we are readily available in between appointments in order to be able to react quickly and adjust medications appropriately when need be. This takes close communication and trust, which is vital to the doctor-patient relationship. I will briefly talk about the antidepressants, and then I will discuss the mood stabilizers that I work with the most.

It is important to note that not all patients who have bipolar disorder need antidepressants, and that in some cases antidepressants may destabilize the mood and drive the person into mania. This is especially the case with Bipolar I Disorder. However, for most patients with bipolar disorder, this is not the case. There is a school of thought among some psychiatrists that antidepressants should not be used for any type of bipolar disorder, but I vehemently disagree with them. I am dedicated to making sure every patient gets to full remission, and in the case of bipolar patients, most have the best results by combining mood stabilizers with antidepressants.

a) **Antidepressants:** I have used all of the different antidepressants that I discussed earlier regarding the treatment of unipolar patients. The first choice is usually between an SNRI and an SSRI, and I make the decision in basically the same way. If the patient tends toward somatic symptoms, anxiety, and depression, or if SSRIs were tried and failed, an SNRI would be the logical choice. If the symptoms are more serotonergic in nature, then an SSRI may be the better choice. Sometimes neither of them is an appropriate choice.

There is a school of thought in the treatment of bipolar disorders that SNRIs should be avoided since they have an increased risk of activation and potential mania. That may be the case with an acute Bipolar I patient, when we need to be careful with any antidepressant; however, for most cases of bipolar disorder, an SNRI is well tolerated if it is the right medication for an individual. An SSRI is more appropriate if there are no obvious noradrenergic symptoms but rather mostly serotonergic symptoms. It is not always easy to tell, so if one is not sure, then it may be best to try one class and then the other to see which is best. I'm looking for the agent that gives only positive results without any significant side effects, which, of course, is the ideal to shoot for. Efficacy of an antidepressant is usually very quick when it comes to treating these patients, even faster than with unipolar disorder, which is already pretty fast. It's exciting to witness these dramatically positive results.

b) **Wellbutrin:** This medication holds a special place for the treatment of bipolar patients. I almost always prescribe Wellbutrin XL since it is very convenient since it is taken once a day, first thing in the morning, and the effect lasts all day. Aplenzin is the newer name-brand version of Wellbutrin XL. If a medication lasts too long and leads to insomnia, then I switch to Wellbutrin SR, and even less likely, Wellbutrin IR. When it comes to the treatment of unipolar disorders, this is not usually a first-line antidepressant but much more likely an augmenting agent. When it comes to treatment of bipolar patients, though, it is more likely than for unipolar disorder to be a first-line choice. The reason is that dopamine is the key neurochemical that is usually imbalanced in these patients, so a boost in the right direction can make a big difference, not just augmentation, which I will discuss next.

I will discuss mood stabilizers next, but the most common ones that I use are the atypical antipsychotics, whose key action is dopamine antagonism and serotonin antagonism. This is good for stabilizing mood, and mood stabilizers may help depression, but they also can lead to the uncovering or worsening of depression. Since Wellbutrin is a dopamine and norepinephrine reuptake inhibitor, it boosts forward dopamine all day, leading to resolution of depression, increased energy, increased motivation and drive, increased sex drive, improved memory, and increased focus. Those with higher-grade bipolar disorder tend to only need and tolerate the lower dose of Wellbutrin XL 150 mg, though some may be in the 300 to 450 mg range. Since the cases that fall within the bipolar spectrum are lower-grade variations, 150 mg may be enough, but they are more likely to need the average dose of 300 mg or higher, as is the case with unipolar disorder. If Wellbutrin works very well but leads to any mood instability, then the mood stabilizer dose may need to be increased, or another may need to be added. If proper mood stabilization leads to fatigue or leads to depression, the Wellbutrin dose may need to be increased until the ideal balance of dopamine is achieved. I refer to this as balancing dopamine 24/7.

I have referred in my first book to the notion of "dopamine daytime/dopamine nighttime" when referring to the combination of an atypical antipsychotic and Wellbutrin, since they can both work together to regulate the flow of dopamine most properly, increasing it when needed and slowing down and stopping it when needed, thus leading to regulation and stabilization of mood. This works well for cyclical depression by attempting to stop the ups and downs and thus even the person out.

In some patients Wellbutrin is too activating and not tolerated, but that can be the case with any other antidepressant, since the body will only tolerate the ones that are actually needed.

Auvelity (dextromethorphan/bupropion SR) is the newest antidepressant and the only new one in several years. It is a mixture of Wellbutrin SR with dextromethorphan, which boosts glutamate as well as modulating serotonin and norepinephrine. It is a very powerful and effective medication for those with treatment-resistant depression. I use this product after Wellbutrin XL, and only if the product doesn't work very well, works and then "poops out" even after maximizing the dose of Wellbutrin XL at 450 mg or Aplenzin at 522 mg. Since Auvelity (dextromethorphan/bupropion SR) is such a powerful anti-depressant, we need to make sure with our bipolar patient that the mood is adequately stabilized if it is employed.

c) **Lamictal (lamotrigine):** This is a unique antidepressant, which is also a mood stabilizer at the same time. It is the only antidepressant that does not work on either serotonin, norepinephrine, or dopamine. I consider it GABAergic, though its actual actions lead to inhibition of glutamate, the key excitatory neurochemical, thus leading to calming of the brain and nervous system. This is a potential first-line treatment for bipolar depression. It is a very safe and reliable choice for all types of bipolar disorder, from high-grade to low-grade. It is the safest if we are concerned about causing instability and activation with one of the more traditional antidepressants.

If the patient has already tried the other classes of antidepressants and either they are not tolerated or they are tolerated but lead to incomplete results and/or side effects, then Lamictal (lamotrigine) can be added. It can be an ideal agent for those suffering with cyclical depression as well as persistent depression, though it does not tend to control the upper pole of bipolar disorder much, though since it is a mood stabilizer, it can not only affect the lower pole but also somewhat stabilize the upper pole. It is the slowest antidepressant, since it can take a few weeks to a couple of months to achieve the desired results, but it is well worth the wait when it works.

d) **Other antidepressants** that I use much more rarely are MAO inhibitors and tricyclic antidepressants; however, we should consider these with more difficult-to-treat patients. Tricyclics are difficult to tolerate at high doses, but at low doses they can be helpful for insomnia, pain, and anxiety. I particularly have seen some good results with MAO inhibitors in tough cases, such as the Emsam patch (selegiline transdernal system) or an oral one such as Nardil (phenelzine) and others. The dietary restrictions are way overblown since most people don't eat high levels of tyramine-rich foods. It's sure nice to have this class in the arsenal.

e) **Augmenting agents** can include Deplin (L-methylfolate), Nuvigil (armodafinil), Provigil (modafinil), Sunosi (solriamfetol). A stimulant is an option if tolerated and does not cause activation or destabilization; it is most appropriate for those with coexisting ADD/ADHD. It's best to treat both when it coexists with bipolar disorder, whether it be type I, type II, or one of the lesser variations, which is most of them.

2) **Mood Stabilizers:** I break this category down into three groups: the "classics," Lithium Carbonate and Depakote; the "atypical" antipsychotics; and the "anti-seizure" class.

a) **The "classic" mood stabilizers** Lithium carbonate and Depakote have been around a long time and are tried and true. They're certainly effective for the right patient, but they are not usually my first-line choice, though many other doctors use them first-line successfully. Lithium carbonate has proven efficacy for patients with suicidal ideation, persistent depression despite trials of antidepressants, and mania with psychotic features, and I have had very good success with certain patients with its use. However, blood monitoring is needed to monitor the level as well as to make sure it does not strain the kidneys and thyroid gland. Lithium carbonate can cause side effects such as hypothyroidism, fatigue, cloudy thinking, and restlessness, as well as others.

Depakote ER (Divalproex Sodium) (the form I prescribe the most) is a very effective mood stabilizer for those who struggle with mania or hypomania, along with problems with anger management. Since I believe that the atypical antipsychotic class are the best first-line products for treating bipolar disorder, I use Depakote as a second- or third-line medication. It has the potential tendency to cause weight gain and fatigue; however, other mood stabilizers can also lead to similar side effects. If weight gain is an issue, then Topamax (topiramate) can be an excellent solution. This product also requires blood monitoring at home, including Depakote levels and LFTs. For more difficult bipolar patients, I may combine two or even three different mood stabilizers at the same time, often from different classes.

b) **The "Atypical" Antipsychotics:** This class of medications is most often my first-line choice for mood stabilization. They're very efficacious and usually well tolerated if the right medication is chosen for the right person. Their main action is dopamine antagonism as well as serotonin antagonism, though some of them have other actions such as dopamine partial agonism as well as serotonin partial agonism, and some have actions on norepinephrine receptors. Their main side effects are sedation, weight gain, akathisia, and others. Lab monitoring is occasionally needed to screen for diabetes and high cholesterol, but more labs are needed for lithium carbonate and Depakote. They each have their unique side effect profile and benefits, so the right atypical needs to be chosen for the specific individual, and it may take trying different ones until we find the perfect fit. They also have antidepressant effects, as other mood stabilizers can tend to do.

  c) **The "antiseizure" class:** The ones I have prescribed include Topamax (topiramate), Trileptal (oxcarbazepine), Lamictal (lamotrigine), Neurontin (gabapentin), and Depakote. Topamax (topiramate) and Neurontin (gabapentin) may not be considered by some to be mood stabilizers, but I have seen definite mood stabilization with some patients with their use. I think of them and others in this class (except Depakote) as the "minor" mood stabilizers. These GABAergic medications are also very helpful for anxiety reduction and somatic symptom reduction. Topamax (topiramate) has the added advantage of being one of the only mood stabilizers that actually leads to weight loss, while others may contribute to some weight gain.

The ideal treatment for bipolar disorder typically involves a combination of one to two antidepressants and one to two mood stabilizers, often totaling three to four medications or more, in order to achieve maximal stability of mood and lead to full remission. Some patients require only one to two medications, while others may need six or more. I usually only prescribe one medication at a time, and my choices are made depending, as I said earlier, on the history, current symptoms, and response to previous medications in the past and currently. I continue augmenting with antidepressants, mood stabilizers, or other supplements when needed, as I follow the course of the illness, with the goal being to achieve a completely stable mood without cycling or mood swings and without recurrence of significant depression, anxiety, mania, or hypomania, and I don't stop until the patient has the correct medication cocktail in order to achieve the best quality of life.

Eating Disorders

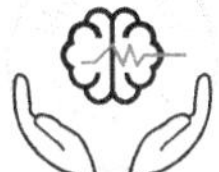

Eating Disorders

This is a very impactful and important topic to discuss. Patients with disordered eating habits are among the most difficult and complex patients to treat. There are so many facets to this disorder, including medical, psychological, and genetic factors; family involvement, including parents and siblings; and irrational thinking, all tied in with underlying mood disorders and addictive behaviors with obsessive thinking about weight and body image. Eating disorders, in my opinion, are really a form of obsessive-compulsive disorder with impulsive thoughts and behaviors, along with frequently an element of bipolar spectrum disorder. Compulsive eating, such as binge eating disorder, which leads to obesity, and bulimia nervosa, as well as the compulsive rejection of food in anorexia nervosa, all have an underlying addictive, obsessive, impulsive, and compulsive component.

I will list the latest DSM-5 diagnostic criteria, followed by my strategic treatment approach. For more information about the subject, I have a long and detailed chapter about it in my first book of the *Healing the Mind and Body* trilogy series, chapter 12, entitled "Eaten Alive by Eating Disorders."

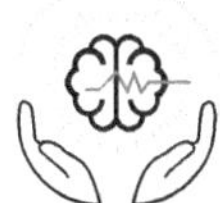

Anorexia Nervosa

1) Restriction of energy intake relative to requirements, leading to a significantly low body weight in the context of age, sex, developmental trajectory, and physical health.

2) Intense fear of gaining weight or becoming fat, or persistent behavior that interferes with weight gain, even though at a significantly low weight.

3) Disturbance in the way in which one's body weight or shape is experienced, undue influence of body weight or shape on self-evaluation, or persistent lack of recognition of the seriousness of the current low body weight.

Not all patients with anorexia nervosa have the same mixture of signs, symptoms, and behaviors. They often struggle with intense preoccupation with their weight and shape. They may weigh themselves frequently, make frequent comments about feeling "fat," have distorted thinking about certain parts of their bodies, and exercise excessively, and the change in weight can have a significant impact on their thinking and behaviors. They tend to spend a lot of time thinking about and preparing their food and tend to have a limited range of what they eat, what they deem as "safe" foods. Their thinking about food is very rigid and difficult to reason with. They may obsessively count calories, and they're especially afraid of fat, having difficulty distinguishing "good fats" from "bad fats." They also may abnormally restrict carbohydrates, meats, processed foods, or whatever they deem as "unhealthy."

Anorexia nervosa is a potentially life-threatening condition, with electrolyte imbalances, cardiac problems, and potential organ failure. While most common among females, it is estimated that about 10 to 15% occurs among males. It happens at all ages, but the peak incidence is definitely in adolescence. It is more common among certain sports, such as gymnastics, cheerleading, dancing (especially ballerinas), wrestling, or any sport where there is a focus on weight. It is also quite common among models, whom these girls unfortunately look up to with regard to body type and body image. It is the third most common chronic illness among adolescents in the United States.

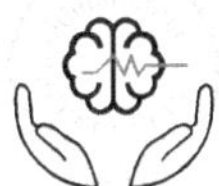

Bulimia Nervosa

A. Recurrent episodes of binge eating.

   1) Eating, in a discrete period of time, an amount of food that is definitely larger than most people would eat during a similar period of time and under similar circumstances.

   2) A sense of lack of control over eating during the episode.

B. Recurrent inappropriate compensatory behavior in order to prevent weight gain, such as self-induced vomiting, misuse of laxatives, diuretics, or other medications; fasting; or extreme exercise.

C. At least once a week for three months.

D. Self-evaluation is unduly influenced by body shape and weight.

Bulimia nervosa is also potentially a dangerous and life-threatening condition, as is anorexia nervosa. There can also be electrolyte imbalances, cardiac problems, problems with other organs, dental problems from corrosion due to the acid from purging, and other medical problems such as acid reflux, irritable bowel syndrome, and other GI complaints. Some have cycles of binging, followed by cycles of dieting, followed by cycles of binging, etc. Overeating and purging tend to coincide with negative mood states, whether depression or even mania. They tend to overuse diet pills and "energy" supplements, and they are also at a higher potential for abusing illicit street stimulants such as cocaine, amphetamines, and methamphetamines. They tend to binge on sugars, carbohydrates, and other high-caloric foods.

One warning sign to watch for is if they leave for the bathroom right after meals. They also secretly binge and purge, more often in the late evening when cravings are often the highest and when other people aren't watching. They often plan ahead for opportunities to binge and purge and often feel a lack of control over eating habits. They're also judgmental and self-critical based on their weight, and there is a high association with mood disorders, from major depressive disorder to anxiety disorders to bipolar disorder to ADD/ADHD and beyond. There is also a significant addictive component, not only associated with the binging, but they also get pleasure and a "high" from purging, as strange as that sounds. They feel in a sense that they get the "best of both worlds" by enjoying the food going in as well as it going out. They enjoy the sense of being in control, though the reality is that the disorder is controlling them.

This is also a very difficult disorder to treat since there are so many components, from medical, psychological, and genetic factors to family dynamics, relationships with family and friends, and an addictive component, as well as mood disorders caused by neurochemical imbalances, all rolled into one.

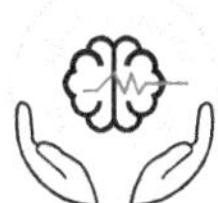

Binge Eating Disorder

A. Recurrent episodes of binge eating. An episode of binge eating is characterized by both of the following:

1. Eating, in a discrete period of time (for example, in any 2-hour period), an amount of food that is definitely larger than most people would eat in a similar period of time under similar circumstances.

2. A sense of lack of control over eating during the episodes (for example, the feeling that one cannot stop eating or control what or how much one is eating).

B. The binge-eating episodes are associated with three (or more) of the following:

- Eating much more rapidly than normal.

- Eating until feeling uncomfortably full.

- Eating large amounts of food when not feeling physically hungry.

- Eating alone because of feeling embarrassed by how much one is eating.

- Feeling disgusted with oneself, depressed, or very guilty afterwards.

- Marked distress regarding binge eating is present.

- The binge eating occurs, on average, at least once a week for three months.

The binge eating is not associated with the recurrent use of inappropriate compensatory behavior (for example, purging) and does not occur excessively during the course of anorexia nervosa, bulimia nervosa, or avoidant/restrictive food intake disorder.

Binge eating disorder can lead to obesity, which also has a lot of medical consequences, such as heart disease, diabetes, high cholesterol, organ dysfunction, and other medical problems. This is also often associated with a lack of an adequate exercise program, over-drinking, smoking, and other unhealthy habits. This, as well as the other eating disorders, is an obsessive, compulsive, impulsive, and addictive behavior. With this and other eating disorders, the person is self-medicating the underlying emotional and psychological aspects, which are the core of the problem. There are also many psychiatric problems associated, from major depressive disorder to bipolar disorder and everywhere in-between.

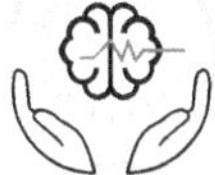

Treatment Strategies

In my opinion, in almost all cases of eating disorders, psychotropic medications are invaluable in order to fully treat and eventually cure these extremely stubborn conditions that plague millions of Americans and also occur throughout the rest of the world. They are much more common in affluent societies where there are many more food choices available and where body image can become an obsession.

Medications alone, though, are usually not enough, since it is imperative to seek psychological help when needed, as well as a nutritionist/dietitian when needed. The team approach is best when treating such stubborn conditions as eating disorders. My focus, of course, is on medications, and thankfully there are so many good choices available at our disposal. However, we cannot ignore the other non-medication factors that are also very important.

A) **SSRIs:** This class is the most classic treatment for eating disorders, since serotonin is often the most important neurochemical involved. All the SSRIs work, but the "classic" one is the first one, Prozac (fluoxetine). Patients with anorexia nervosa tend to need lower-to-average doses, such as 10 to 20 mg or so, while patients with bulimia nervosa tend to need higher doses, such as the classic 60 mg dose, in the 40 to 80 mg range. However, they may only need more average doses, and anorexics may need higher doses, depending on the individual. All the SSRIs work, but I have tended toward Prozac (fluoxetine), Lexapro (escitalopram), Zoloft (sertraline), Viibryd (vilazodone), and Trintellix (vortioxetine). Since SSRIs are the classic treatment for OCD, it makes sense that they are also for eating disorders, since it is basically an obsessive-compulsive problem. For some, serotonin is the only significant neurochemical imbalance, but that is not the norm. Most likely augmentation and sometimes switching to a better first-line agent will be needed in order to achieve our treatment goals.

B) **SNRIs:** I'm sure you know by now that I'm a big fan of this class. It's definitely the most common medication class that I prescribe first-line, especially if there are significant somatic and/or anxiety symptoms associated, which just so happens to be most of the time. In a significant amount of ED patients this class will be better than the SSRIs, though SSRIs are still very good for many. Since mood disorders are often comorbid with other mood disorders and medical problems, more complete balancing of the neurochemicals may be better than those with only single action. It really just depends if norepinephrine is a significant component of the overall picture or not.

Since serotonin is the most important neurochemical involved in eating disorders, this is why SSRIs are such a successful treatment. If one is not sure, it doesn't hurt to try one class and then the other separately and see for ourselves which is the better choice. Sometimes comparing medications in the same class, whether SNRIs or SSRIs, is necessary in order to see which gives the best results with the least side effects.

Pristiq (desvenlafaxine) is my favorite in this class, followed by Effexor XR (venlafaxine ER), but Cymbalta (duloxetine) and Fetzima (levomilnacipran) are also very good choices for some. Fetzima (levomilnacipran) has a 2:1 ratio of norepinephrine to serotonin, so it can be helpful in some of the more somatic and highly anxious patients, which is fine as long as it is not too noradrenergic, which can cause activation and nervousness in some. Cymbalta (duloxetine) is more even between the two, a bit more serotonergic than the others, which may cause fatigue and nausea in some. Pristiq (desvenlafaxine) and Effexor XR (venlafaxine ER) seem to have the ideal ratio between serotonin and norepinephrine for many, leading to well-balanced and overall well-tolerated results. However, as I said, they are all good. The important point is which one is better for which individual, which of course is found out during the rational trial-and-error approach.

C) **Wellbutrin:** This medication is a bit controversial when it comes to treating EDs, especially when treating anorexia nervosa or bulimia nervosa. There is a concern that it may increase the risk of seizures, which is a valid concern if one is dealing with an active disorder, due to electrolyte imbalances and other unhealthy physical changes. If one has recovered, however, from the active phase of the disorder and is in remission, then it may be appropriate and sometimes even necessary to add Wellbutrin in order to achieve the most complete results. If I'm concerned, I can easily check a full lab panel, including, of course, electrolytes (especially potassium but also the others) and organ function first and make sure the person is medically healthy, but if dopamine is imbalanced, there is no better medication to block the abnormal reuptake of dopamine and norepinephrine and increase their flow throughout the day than Wellbutrin. I usually prescribe the XL form, since it lasts the longest and only needs to be taken once a day, first thing in the morning. The shorter-acting SR version may be better for some if the longer-acting form lasts too long.

Auvelity (dextromethorphan/bupropion SR) is the newest antidepressant that combines Wellbutrin SR with dextromethorphan, which mainly boosts glutamate, the main excitatory neurochemical, but also modulates serotonin and norepinephrine. This combined effect leads to very powerful results. It is certainly an exciting medication to work with when we are dealing with treatment-resistant depression. I reach for the samples when Wellbutrin XL doesn't work very well or when it does work well but then the positive effects "poop out" even with increasing Wellbutrin XL to the maximum dose of 450 mg or Aplenzin 522 mg.

I refer to dopamine as the "pleasure" chemical or the "sex, drugs, and rock 'n' roll" neurochemical since balancing dopamine can lead to increased energy, joy, motivation, drive, passion for life, focus, concentration, memory, sex drive, and sexual functioning. I consider Wellbutrin to be a significant "quality of life" medication, which is why it is my favorite augmenting agent in order to get the patient closer to and even able to achieve complete remission.

D) **Topamax (topiramate):** This is my other favorite augmenting agent, which is a very unique medication that primarily works on improving the flow of GABA, which leads to relaxation of the nervous system. It's always best to think preventatively and not just reactively. GABA is the main inhibitory neurochemical, which leads to a calming effect on the brain and nervous system as well as many other nice surprises. I certainly wouldn't give it to an anorexic patient; however, it is very useful for bulimic patients as well as those with binge eating disorder. It has a unique effect of reducing the cravings for sugars and carbohydrates, the very foods that they tend to binge on. When the cravings go down, the binging goes down as well; thus, this gives the patient some semblance of control over a disorder when it's difficult to achieve that. They then tend more toward proteins, vegetables, and fruits, foods that are least likely to be purged.

Since more binging occurs in the afternoon to evening, the generic version is often best timed when taken an hour or more before cravings and binging would normally start. Since this is an odd time to take a medication and may be difficult to remember, I advise my patients to set an alarm on their phone that goes off every day as a reminder. If one of the longer-acting versions like Trokendi XR or Qudexy XR (topiramate ER) is used, then I usually give it in the morning, since it lasts all day and evening, while the shorter-acting version may wear off after half a day, necessitating taking it twice a day for some who binge daytime and nighttime. They're all highly effective, though, so it comes down to which is more available, which is less expensive, and whichever the patient prefers when given the choice. As I said, I usually give the short-acting form because I have had a lot of experience and success with it.

This medication also is excellent for not only prevention of migraine headaches, for which it is classically known to work and for which it is even FDA-approved, but also for "off-label" reduction of many other somatic symptoms throughout the body. It also works very well for anxiety prevention, due to the improved balance of GABA and thus an overall relaxing effect on the mind and body during the day and in the evening, and it can also be helpful for sleep quality. Part of why tranquilizers like benzodiazepines and sleeping pills reduce anxiety is that they temporarily balance GABA, along with their tranquilizing effects, though the GABAergic medications such as Topamax (topiramate), Neurontin (gabapentin), Trileptal (oxcarbazepine), Tegretol (carbamazepine), Keppra (levetiracetam), Depakote, and others preventatively balance GABA, thus leading to prevention of anxiety and somatic symptoms before they would occur in the first place.

E) **Lamictal (lamotrigine)** is also included in this family but is different since its strength is bipolar depression, cyclical depression, and other variations that are more difficult to treat. It is a very unique medication that is the slowest one I work with, but when it works, it is worth the wait. It not only gets the person out of depression but also keeps them there over the long haul. It may affect the upper pole, but its strength is the lower pole. It's certainly nice to have so many great options in this very impactful class of medications.

F) **The Atypicals:** The atypical antipsychotic class is another of my favorites to prescribe, especially for those patients that are more difficult and complex to treat, which certainly describes ED patients. Some of them have a definite bipolar component, with mania and hypomania, while many present more subtly, such as persistent depression, recurrent depression, cyclical depression, treatment-resistant depression, atypical depression, or any other individual that does not fully respond to antidepressants alone when we think they should. The main action of atypicals is dopamine and serotonin antagonism, some with agonist effects on serotonin and/or dopamine, as well as others with effects on norepinephrine. This variety of mechanisms of action leads to some excellent choices with different individual responses.

Wellbutrin speeds up dopamine, while the atypicals calm it down. This is why I often combine them for a "dopamine daytime-dopamine nighttime" effect, balancing dopamine 24/7. Risperdal (risperidone) was the atypical I prescribed to treat EDs early on and is a decent medication, but it can cause fatigue, weight gain, and rarely hyperprolactinemia (causing milk discharge from the breasts). Weight gain can be good for anorexic patients, as long as they are able to handle the weight gain psychologically. Zyprexa (olanzapine) would be good if weight gain is needed, but often the weight gain is too much and the person is not able to handle that amount psychologically. Abilify (aripiprazole) is a very good medication and usually well tolerated, though weight gain can be problematic for some. Seroquel (quetiapine) and Seroquel XR (quetiapine ER) are excellent medications but may be too sedating for some.

The newer medications in this class are Saphris (asenapine), Latuda (lurasidone), Rexulti (brexpiprazole), Vraylar (cariprazine), Caplyta (lumateperone), Fanapt (iloperidone) (which has been available for several years as a treatment for schizophrenia but more recently has gotten the indication for bipolar disorder and is metabolically friendly with a low risk of weight gain), and Lybalvi (olanzapine and samidorphan) (which is basically Zyprexa (olanzapine) combined with a component that prevents some of the weight gain seen with Zyprexa (olanzapine), which has been its biggest weakness). Latuda (lurasidone) is one of the atypicals that is more metabolically friendly, thus useful for patients who are bulimic, binge eaters, or obese or for those who really don't want to gain weight. It is also generic and thus less expensive. The good news for some, though, is that for this issue, Topamax (topiramate) can be the answer that the patient is looking for.

Weight can be followed easily enough, along with checking glucose to screen for the development and worsening of diabetes, as well as cholesterol, thyroid function studies, a chemistry panel including kidney and liver function and electrolytes such as potassium and sodium, and other necessary labs. This medication class is invaluable when it comes to fully treating patients who are more difficult and complex and so desperately need to be treated in the right way.

G) **Other augmenting choices** could be Deplin (L-methylfolate) (a high-quality folic acid supplement that increases the production of serotonin, norepinephrine, and dopamine), Nuvigil (armodafinil), Provigil (modafinil), and Sunosi (solriamfetol). Nuvigil (armodafinil) and Provigil (modafinil) boost dopamine and histamine, while Sunosi (solriamfetol) is a DNRI, thus boosting dopamine and norepinephrine. These actions provide the energizing effects. They work well for persistent fatigue, residual depression, ADD, and fatigue associated with sleep apnea and are helpful for shift workers who work the graveyard shift in order to recreate the feeling of daytime during working hours. Even stimulants may be needed, as long as they are tolerated and safe for the individual, except for the anorexic patients, of course.

There are other supplements and pharmaceutical medications that can be added to suit the needs of the individual, since we need to use whatever it takes in order to achieve our goal of complete remission for every patient. Eating disorders can certainly be difficult to treat, but it is well worth the effort in the end when we see the results that lead to our goal of remission and complete stability of life.

CHAPTER SIX

ADD/ADHD

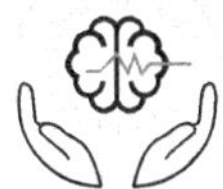

CHAPTER SIX

ADD/ADHD

Attention Deficit Disorder/Attention Deficit Hyperactivity Disorder is a disorder noted for a trio of symptoms: inattention, hyperactivity, and impulsivity. This disorder arises in part from abnormalities in various circuits involving the prefrontal cortex. There are a variety of ways that people who have this disorder present, some hyperactive as children and adults and some not, some with impulsivity problems and some without, and other individual variations. Inattention, though, is an issue with all, children or adults. In adults it can be referred to as executive dysfunction, which refers to the inability to sustain attention and thus the ability to solve problems.

The reason that individuals develop this condition is due to genetic predisposition. Either the mother or father has it, possibly both, as well as siblings and other family members. In previous generations it was less likely to have been diagnosed and treated. It is not uncommon that when it is identified in a child, I then see parents and siblings for the same. With what I do for a living, I see a lot of dramatic changes when I treat adults for a variety of conditions such as depression, anxiety, and bipolar disorder, as well as all of the other mood disorders that I discuss in this and all of my other books. However, it is difficult to match the dramatic changes that we see so quickly when we treat adults with ADD. They often reflect about how different their lives would have been had they been treated properly when they were younger. I share with them that we cannot do anything about the past, but rather we can be grateful that this will change their future. It should not be a surprise that this is a genetic problem, since that is the case with pretty much all of the diagnoses related to neurochemical imbalances.

There are a variety of other symptoms besides difficulty with focus and concentration. These include easy distractibility, difficulty staying on task and completing tasks, difficulty organizing, difficulty multitasking, racing thoughts (though this could also be from bipolar disorder or an anxiety disorder), interrupting others, decreased memory, losing things easily, difficulty being on time, difficulty reading, reckless driving, reckless behaviors, and an increased risk of drug abuse.

Common comorbid conditions include depression, anxiety disorders, bipolar disorders, eating disorders, and others. For more details about this common and disabling disorder, see my first and third books of the *Healing the Mind and Body* trilogy series.

Another symptom of ADHD is *selective* inattention. For example, if a parent asks me why his or her son has no difficulty at all focusing on video games and his iPhone but has difficulty doing social studies, english, or math homework, I tell them that the reason is that he enjoys doing the former but does not enjoy doing the latter. An adult may have no difficulty making a sale but dreads sitting at his desk catching up with emails and calls and doing paperwork. If the person really enjoys what he or she is doing, then it is easier to focus and concentrate, while if an activity is not enjoyable or interesting, then the attention can tend to wane.

ADD/ADHD has nothing to do with intelligence. It has everything to do with the inability to be able to show one's true potential. Many people with this disorder are quite intelligent but are unable to tap into that potential on a regular basis due to something that is not their fault and not within their control. He or she may be labeled as smart but lazy or a dreamer.

One of the problems with not treating it is reduced self-esteem and confidence. Also, the person may not be achieving his or her true potential, which can be discouraging and depressing. This also leads to an increased risk of addiction by self-medicating and other areas of dysfunction in life. Treatment of this disorder is dramatic and extremely impactful to the patient, who is often amazed at the difference in life. We will discuss the specifics regarding treatments a little later on.

ADHD/ADD has traditionally been considered a childhood disorder, but we also recognize that it is very common in adults. There can be different features in children than in adults, though both share many common features, which really depends on the individuality of the person. Nevertheless, the "classic" form of ADHD has the onset by the age of seven to twelve years old. There is a lot of variability, though, since some have more symptoms in childhood than others. You can tell some kids even by the age of three to four years old, while some don't have significant symptoms until later in life. Some people may get by with their natural intelligence and work ethic until a certain point when the curriculum gets more difficult, such as from middle school to high school to college to grad school, which is more common as one's education advances, getting progressively more difficult each step of the way.

Some who did not present as hyperactive may have more easily slipped through the cracks, since the hyperactive and impulsive kids get all the attention. The inattentive kids, which in my experience is the most common presentation, tend to tune out, stare out the window, daydream, and doodle, while not really hearing what the teacher is saying and not really caring. Kids and adults with ADD/ADHD tend to be bored easily and do just what is needed to get by but nothing extra. They can quite easily move through the school system without recognizing the difficulty with focus, concentration, and attention. Since they're doing "well enough," they just may get pushed through the school system (especially the public school system) and workplace without much fanfare. They may never achieve their true potential, which is sad, since the treatment is quite simple and effective.

The hyperactive and impulsive kids tend to get the attention and may not be getting the attention needed or get the wrong kind of attention. However, hyperactivity declines notably by adolescence and early adulthood, though some remain that way. Treating a hyperactive kid with a stimulant doesn't make sense initially at first glance, until you understand how it works and what it does.

Proper education of the parents not only benefits the children, but it also may uncover it in at least one of the parents, which can lead to further treatment when needed, thus leading to a better home environment for everyone. Parents are often hesitant about giving any medications to their kids, who they perceive as too young to warrant such treatment, or they think the kid is just being lazy and not trying hard enough. Some feel that giving stimulants to kids is like giving them meth, and then they will become addicts because of treating this condition.

I don't like to discriminate whom I treat based on age. If the parent wouldn't have difficulty treating their kid with diabetes, why should that medical problem be any different than this medical problem? Even adults are often hesitant to treat, since they may just think that is the way they are, and it is just normal for them. Some doctors may be hesitant to treat an adult who has a history of addiction, and I will discuss this controversial topic a bit later when I discuss treatment options.

The prevalence in adults may be only about half of that in children, but it is also not recognized as easily and thus tends to go untreated, or the adult may treat it with caffeine and other stimulants. Whereas half of all children and adolescents with ADHD are thought to be diagnosed and treated, less than one in five adults with ADHD is thought to be diagnosed and treated. There is also a lot of comorbidity with mood disorders. I believe that at least 10% of the population has some variation of ADD/ADHD. It is one of the most underrecognized and undertreated conditions that we face as providers. Proper treatment most often leads to a dramatic improvement of quality of life and can even save lives. Before we talk about treatment, though, I will list the DSM-5 criteria for ADD/ADHD.

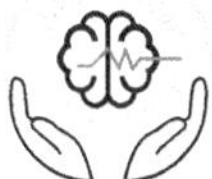

DSM-5 Criteria for ADD/ADHD

ADHD/ADD is a persistent pattern of inattention and/or hyperactivity-impulsivity that interferes with functioning or development, has symptoms presenting in two or more settings (e.g., at home, school, or work; with friends or relatives; in other activities), and negatively impacts directly on social, academic, or occupational functioning. Several symptoms must have been present before age 12 years.

- A persistent pattern of inattention and/or hyperactivity-impulsivity that interferes with functioning or development.

- Six or more of the symptoms have persisted for at least six months to a degree that is inconsistent with developmental level and that negatively impacts directly ly on social and academic/occupational activities. **Please note:** The symptoms are not solely a manifestation of oppositional behavior, defiance, hostility, or failure to understand tasks or instructions. For older adolescents and adults (age 17 or older), five or more symptoms are required.

- Several inattentive or hyperactive-impulsive symptoms were present prior to age 12 years.

- Several inattentive or hyperactive-impulsive symptoms are present in two or more settings (e.g., at home, school, or work; with friends or relatives; in other activities).

- There is clear evidence that the symptoms interfere with, or reduce the quality of, social, academic, or occupational functioning.

- The symptoms do not occur exclusively during the course of schizophrenia or another psychotic disorder and are not better explained by another mental disorder (e.g., a mood disorder, anxiety disorder, dissociative disorder, personality disorder, substance intoxication, or withdrawal).

While the fundamental diagnostic criteria for ADHD have not changed in the DSM-5 as compared to the DSM-IV, there is more attention to more accurately characterizing the experience of adolescents and adults with ADHD. Adults and adolescents are required to present with a minimum of five (rather than six) symptoms, and symptoms should have been present before age 12 (not before age 7), recognizing that adult recall of precise childhood onset is difficult. A pervasive developmental disorder like Autistic Spectrum Disorder is no longer an exclusion criterion. ADHD is now listed in the new category of neurodevelopmental disorder, acknowledging the growing body of scientific evidence supporting the fact that brain development correlates with ADHD. Although motor symptoms of hyperactivity become less obvious in adolescence and adulthood, difficulty persists with restlessness, inattention, poor planning, and impulsivity. A substantial proportion of children remain relatively impaired into adulthood, and as I said previously, this disorder is extremely underrecognized and undertreated. Hopefully that will change in the near future.

Individuals with ADHD may present with both inattention and hyperactivity/impulsivity, or one symptom pattern may predominate. The three presentations of ADHD are commonly referred to as combined-type, inattentive-type, and hyperactive/impulsive-type. According to the DSM-5 classification system, the appropriate presentation of ADHD should be indicated based on the predominant symptom pattern for the last six months. Furthermore, it must be specified whether the individual with ADHD is in "partial remission"—when fewer than the full ADHD criteria have been met for the past six months, but symptoms still result in impairment in social, academic, or occupational functioning—and the current severity of the disease. There are also mild, moderate, and severe presentations, as is the case with any disorder related to neurochemical imbalances.

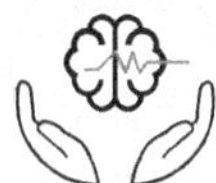

Treatment of ADD/ADHD

ADHD patients generally cannot activate prefrontal cortex areas appropriately in response to cognitive tasks of attention and executive functioning. This is because dopamine and norepinephrine dysregulation in ADHD prevents the normal "tuning" of neurons in the prefrontal cortex. One problem is that the forward firing of norepinephrine and dopamine through the brain is too slow, preventing the optimal downstream benefits. The other problem can be leakage of the presynaptic neuron sites at norepinephrine and dopamine, causing an abnormal backflow of the chemicals the wrong way. ADHD is really thus a two-pronged problem, meaning that the electricity and plumbing both need to be fixed.

Certain drugs, such as the street stimulants, especially hijack the dopamine system, leading to uncontrolled dopamine firing that reinforces the reward of drug abuse and leads to compulsive behaviors such as mindless self-destructive drug-seeking behaviors. I have referred to dopamine as the "pleasure chemical" or the "sex, drugs, and rock 'n roll" chemical. Thus, fine-tuning the dopamine reward pathway can lead to true happiness and joy. Improving the flow of norepinephrine and dopamine in the brain is vitally important if it is needed, since the quality of life of the individual depends on it.

The development of drug and alcohol abuse, impulsivity, inattention, and anxiety are all comorbid with ADHD, particularly in adolescents and adults. It is also important to note that the timing of the onset of ADHD suggests that the formation of synapses, and especially the selection of synapses, may explain why the prevalence of ADHD in adults is only half that in children and adolescents. It may not only be associated with an imbalance of norepinephrine or dopamine but also output to alpha-2A adrenergic receptors as well as serotonin receptors, GABA receptors, and some other problems that are under active investigation. Associated factors that lead to an increased risk of ADHD include preterm birth, maternal smoking during pregnancy, addictions, etc.

Inattentive symptoms are not really seen in preschool children with ADHD, perhaps because they do not have a sufficiently mature prefrontal cortex to manifest this symptom in a manner that is abnormal compared to normal development. Most studies of stimulants involve children over the age of six, though they may be appropriate in kids under that age if needed and if tolerated. Once inattention becomes a prominent symptom of ADHD, it remains so over the person's entire life. However, hyperactivity declines notably by adolescence and early adulthood, while the recognized comorbidities I mentioned skyrocket in frequency as ADD patients enter adulthood. This condition doesn't just treat itself, which is where we come in. If we don't treat them, then they will tend to treat themselves. Our methods are better and safer than theirs are, and we can prove that to them.

A) **Stimulants:** These are the "gold standard" treatment strategy that cannot be matched with regard to efficacy. The issue has to do with tolerance and appropriateness depending on the patient. Since there is so much coexistence with mood disorders, I tend to treat them first before I treat the ADD/ADHD, depending on the situation, of course. Antidepressants and mood stabilizers can help to treat core ADD/ADHD symptoms, and in some cases that is all that is needed. If ADHD predominates, then we can always start with a stimulant and then augment from there. In more complex cases, however, it is important to treat the underlying addictions and mood disorders that may predominate, making treatment more difficult since we usually need to wait until sobriety is achieved and maintained and it is safe to proceed. Once the underlying addictions and coexisting mood disorders are adequately treated, and if there are still significant ADHD symptoms, then we can focus on that aspect and "fine-tune" the treatment with the goal of complete remission in mind.

Stimulants serve two purposes: to stimulate the neurochemicals to move forward fast enough to optimally connect within the brain, especially norepinephrine and dopamine. The other action is to slightly inhibit the reuptake of norepinephrine and dopamine at the presynaptic cell membrane. They do not do this though as well as the non-stimulants that I will mention next. Since ADD/ADHD often travels with depression, anxiety, bipolar disorder, and other mood disorders, a combination of a stimulant with non-stimulants in order to deal with each problem separately is the best method in order to achieve the most complete and satisfying results.

Treating all of these comorbid disorders together is always the best approach, since incomplete treatment leads to incomplete and inadequate results. ADHD may be considered as an afterthought since the mood disorders often predominate and demand immediate attention. It should be more of a focus than it is (no pun intended), since resolving ADD symptoms so markedly improves quality of life. This may explain why the polypharmaceutical approach is the rule and not the exception when following the Corona Protocol. Since lack of comorbidity in adults with ADD is not as common. This explains why the majority of adults with this condition are not adequately treated, as is the case with coexisting mood disorders.

The surprising and quite amazing feature about stimulants is that they actually have a calming effect on those who have ADHD. They tend to reduce anxiety and calm the brain, which doesn't make sense at first glance since they are stimulants. However, that is one way to know if ADD/ADHD is being treated properly, regarding whether the mind is calmer or is overstimulated. If there is overstimulation but good results regarding treatment of ADHD, then this may be a signal to lower the dose or to augment with a mood stabilizer and/or an antidepressant quickly in order to stabilize the mood. If mood stabilization or treatment of anxiety and depressive disorders is already completed, then it may be time to add a stimulant to treat the continued ADHD symptoms. This can improve energy and motivation in some, but some patients have residual fatigue and decreased motivation requiring augmentation, thus achieving a mixture of antidepressants and stimulants in order to get the best of both worlds.

Combining ADHD medications with atypical antipsychotics is also a very impactful treatment for certain individuals. The trick is to not increase the mania or psychotic thinking with stimulants while at the same time not over-sedating with mood stabilizers and causing depressive symptoms with reduced energy, motivation, and drive as well as increased ADD symptoms. The atypicals inhibit dopamine, while the stimulants and Wellbutrin increase its forward flow during the daytime, thus balancing dopamine 24/7 when combining two competing dopamine agents, which can work together in a symbiotic fashion in order to achieve the best therapeutic results.

The controversial subject that I alluded to earlier is what to do with a patient who has a history of addiction. How to proceed really depends on the situation. If alcohol, benzos, opiates, or others comprise the addiction history, then it is probably okay to treat the ADD once the addiction and underlying mood disorders are attended to. I do not believe that if someone has an addictive history, it is always unwise to prescribe controlled substances. Some take the approach that all controlled substances are to be avoided with any addict, but it's really not that simple.

Even in the case of those who were addicted to methamphetamines, cocaine, or even prescription stimulants, they may properly be treated with stimulants if the patient is in sobriety from the previous substances and if the patient is followed closely and attention is paid to the individual's response to treatment while paying close attention to try to avoid relapse. We can give limited quantities when we start treatment, and we can keep a close eye on the CURES reports to make sure the patient is not "doctor shopping." If we are suspicious and have just cause, then we can always do random drug testing to make sure that they are not using anything from the street.

If the person is free from the previous addictions, but the underlying disorder is left untreated, then it is, in my view, more likely that the patient will self-medicate if not treated properly. I would rather try to medicate properly and try to thus decrease the risk of the patient falling back into addiction rather than under-treating, which leads to inadequate functioning in life for that individual. In these patients it is important to treat the ADD, as well as the addiction if it's an issue, along with the underlying mood disorders all at the same time, which leads to the most optimal functioning and quality of life.

Treating the ADD may increase anxiety, mania, and psychotic thinking, which means stopping the stimulant and switching to a mood stabilizer. On the other hand, once mood is adequately stabilized, the addition of a stimulant can be very well-tolerated and have impactful results. Some people are at higher risk for addiction, and thus in these cases optimization of non-stimulants may be the best option, which I will discuss next. Most cases, however, are not that complex and respond quite well to the proper treatment at the proper time.

There are two main classes of ADHD medications, the methylphenidate class and the amphetamine class. They both act as stimulants and also reduce the reuptake of norepinephrine and dopamine, much like the antidepressants do, though they do so much more strongly. The methylphenidate tends to influence norepinephrine a bit more than dopamine, while the amphetamine class focuses less on norepinephrine and more on dopamine, though they are both very effective treatments. The right one depends on the individual. There are way too many stimulants on the market, name-brand and generic. There are more stimulants available than any other class of medications by far.

Whether to use a long-acting versus a short-acting stimulant really just depends on the specific needs of the individual. The reason that longer-acting agents may be better is because of the consistency of the results throughout the day and early evening as well as a decreased risk of addiction. However, the addiction rate is low if ADD/ADHD is diagnosed and treated correctly. The shorter-acting options, though, are more convenient for someone who may take a different amount depending on the day, such as in the case of college or graduate students and people who have short shifts at work.

B) **Strattera (atomoxetine) and Qelbree (viloxazine):** These are unique medications and the only two in this class of NRIs, which are mostly norepinephrine reuptake inhibitors with minimal effect on dopamine. Strattera (atomoxetine) has been generic for many years. More recently the second NRI to be released is Qelbree (viloxazine). Though their main action is norepinephrine reuptake inhibition, they both also slightly use dopamine, and Qelbree (viloxazine) also slightly uses serotonin. My experience with Qelbree (viloxazine) at the time of this writing is limited, but it is certainly nice to have a new option available in our armamentarium. My experience, though, is that an NRI does not work as well as a stimulant, which is still the gold standard when it comes to treatment of ADD/ADHD.

Possibly part of the problem with the non-stimulants is that they mainly work on norepinephrine with a lesser effect on dopamine, which is one of the two most important neurochemicals when it comes to ADD/ADHD. Despite that, though, they just don't have the "punch" of a stimulant. This is not my first-line choice since the stimulants are usually more effective. However, for the right person, these medications can be excellent choices, especially if norepinephrine is the key component of the overall imbalance.

The reason why I don't use this more is because I often use SNRIs since often serotonin is a component of the overall imbalance. If serotonin is not a factor but norepinephrine is, then Strattera (atomoxetine) or Qelbree (viloxazine) would be better choices than an SNRI. It really just depends on the individual presentation of that patient.

Since norepinephrine is also involved in anxiety and somatic symptoms, these NRI medications can also have other benefits than just treating ADD. This medication can work very well for someone who does not tolerate stimulants or where stimulants are contraindicated, such as with certain cardiac problems, a high risk of addiction, or another complicating factor. Even though they are not stimulants, they can work surprisingly well for the right patient. They can be quite beneficial for noradrenergic symptoms, which include improved mood, reduced anxiety, and fewer somatic symptoms. They can also be combined with Wellbutrin and/or stimulants in order to treat each neurochemical most optimally in order to achieve the best results for the inattentive kids.

C) **Wellbutrin:** This medication, along with the newer name-brand Aplenzin, is totally unique since bupropion serves as a weaker or presynaptic reuptake inhibitor of norepinephrine than dopamine; thus, it is an nDRI. This is an amazing medication and is the most common augmenting medication I prescribe. Since dopamine is the "pleasure" chemical, I add this when we need to increase energy and motivation, improve metabolism with weight loss if needed, and increase drive, focus and concentration, memory, sex drive, and sexual functioning, along with increased joy, happiness, and pleasure, as well as treat underlying depression, of course. It can also be the primary treatment for ADD, especially if the patient does not tolerate a stimulant. There are also patients that are successfully treated with stimulants that have residual motivation, fatigue, and possibly depressed mood. In these cases this can be an excellent augmenting agent and can also boost the effectiveness of the stimulant.

Nicotine addiction can be a problem with these patients, since nicotine subjectively improves dopamine release, and this enhances arousal, so it is not surprising that Wellbutrin can be an extremely useful addition to help people beat this destructive habit. For this purpose, bupropion comes in a distant second place to Chantix.

I often add this to ADD medications, since the stimulants only slightly inhibit the reuptake of norepinephrine and dopamine, while Wellbutrin does a much better job of that without actually being a stimulant. It has stimulating effects, so we need to watch for side effects such as increased anxiety, instability of mood, and over-activation in general.

Even if it is not tolerated at one point, that does not mean that it may not be helpful at some later point, especially when mood stabilization has already occurred. Since mood stabilizers can be a bit sedating, it is very helpful to be able to add Wellbutrin XL in order to balance dopamine 24/7.

Adding Wellbutrin can dramatically improve quality of life, and full remission is often achieved with its addition. I prescribe Wellbutrin XL much more than Wellbutrin SR since it is a true once-a-day instead of a twice-a-day medication. If increasing the dose helps the daytime results but leads to instability of mood, then a mood stabilizer can be increased in order to compensate. If the mood stabilizer needs to go higher, which leads to daytime fatigue and lack of motivation, then increasing the dose of Wellbutrin often leads to the results we are seeking. Fine-tuning the antidepressants and mood stabilizers along with ADD medications is the true art and science of rational psychopharmacology.

D) **SNRIs:** The fact that depression and anxiety disorders coexist frequently with ADD/ADHD and the fact that the SNRI is the best overall first-line treatment for depression and anxiety disorders mean it should thus be a frequent choice for these patients. If norepinephrine is imbalanced, it is likely also that serotonin is imbalanced at the same time, which is why an SNRI is often a better choice than Strattera (atomoxetine) or an SSRI, or a combination of the two. If serotonin is not a significant factor, though, then Strattera (atomoxetine), Qelbree (viloxazine), and Wellbutrin may be better choices. This class is also better for those with somatic symptoms, which are frequently undiagnosed as related to the patient's mood. This medication class reduces anxiety and somatic symptoms as well as improves overall mood. If that leads to fatigue, lack of motivation, and residual depression, then the addition of Wellbutrin to bolster dopamine is likely the next augmenting choice. If noradrenergic side effects are problematic, then I would switch to a non-noradrenergic agent such as an SSRI.

E) **Alpha-2A adrenergic agonists:** Alpha-2A receptors are thought to be the primary mediators of the effects of norepinephrine in the prefrontal cortex, regulating symptoms of inattention, hyperactivity, and impulsivity in ADHD. This class can work well with the NRIs Strattera (atomoxetine) and Qelbree (viloxazine) as well as Wellbutrin, SNRIs, and stimulants. This class tends to work well for children and adults with high impulsivity and behavioral problems, as well as insomnia and other negative symptoms affected by primary treatment of the ADHD. There are two direct-acting agonists for alpha-2 receptors used to treat ADHD: guanfacine and clonidine.

Guanfacine is relatively more selective for alpha-2A receptors and is also available in a once-a-day version in the evening called Intuniv (guanfacine hydrochloride), which is the top medication I prescribe in this class. Clonidine is relatively non-selective against alpha-2 receptors. In addition, clonidine has actions on imidazoline receptors, thought to be responsible for some of its sedating and hypotensive actions. I have had a very good experience, however, with both medications, so the decision about which one depends on the individual. However, since guanfacine is more selective and has fewer potential side effects than clonidine, I most often choose it first.

Clonidine is approved for the treatment of hypertension but is "off-label" for the treatment of ADHD. Intuniv (guanfacine hydrochloride) is indicated for ADHD for children but not for adults, though it also works well off-label for adults. This should not matter at all, since off-label means cutting-edge medicine at its best. One of these can be a very good potential addition if full ADHD treatment results are not realized with the other more first-line agents, though it may be a solo agent less often.

F) **Other choices** include Nuvigil (armodafinil), Provigil (modafinil), and Sunosi (solriamfetol), which are non-stimulants but have proven efficacy in the treatment of ADHD, not just for augmentation for depression and chronic fatigue. Basically Nuvigil (armodafinil) and Provigil (modafinil) boost dopamine primarily but also histamine, while Sunosi (solriamfetol) is a DNRI, with its main effect on dopamine and a lesser effect on norepinephrine. They are classically known to be used for fatigue related to sleep apnea, as well as for shift workers that work the graveyard shift, those with chronic fatigue, or those with residual depressive symptoms. They may be effective for those who do not tolerate stimulants or, more likely, as an augmenting agent when there are still residual symptoms.

Deplin (L-methylfolate) may help since it is a folic acid supplement that can increase the production and thus the quantity of serotonin, norepinephrine, and dopamine, so it may be worth a shot, especially if there are also residual depressive symptoms and fatigue.

There used to be a prescription omega-3 fatty acid called Vayarin, though it is no longer available in the United States. This class of supplements, though, can obviously be found over the counter. Other supplements may also be helpful for some, and of course a healthy diet and a regular cardiovascular exercise program can be helpful, as is the case with all mood disorders and other manifestations of neurochemical imbalances. Biofeedback, counseling, and working with an ADD code can be helpful to a person. However, I consider these as supplemental to the gold standard treatment with stimulants as well as all of the other choices that I have discussed in this chapter.

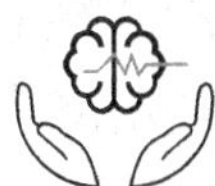

Summary

As you can see, it is very difficult to try to pick apart all of the different types of mood disorders and other manifestations of neurochemical imbalances, since they often combine. Comorbidity is the rule rather than the exception when it comes to all of the various manifestations that we are presented with. If one has different diagnoses, then I pick the most important diagnosis to start with first, and then I attend to each one after that in order of importance.

Another approach is to try to treat two or three of the disorders at the same time with the same medication. An example is someone with depression, anxiety, and somatic symptoms. An SNRI may treat all three at the same time, though it is most likely that augmentation will still be needed. Some medications make some diagnoses better while making others worse at the same time, necessitating fine-tuning in order to achieve the proper balance. The average patient is best treated with two to three medications at the same time. Some need only a solo agent, while some require four to six or more in order to achieve full remission.

Medications only go so far, though, since some people have personality disorders that medications do not treat, while others need psychological counseling instead or, more likely, in addition. Some may need to learn relaxation techniques and coping skills, while others benefit from contemplative prayer, meditation, yoga, massage, acupuncture, physical therapy, chiropractic, or other palliative treatments in order to treat the body, mind, and spirit. The best treatment approach is to individualize and tailor the treatment to suit all the needs so that our patients are happy and healthy and high on life.

www.ingramcontent.com/pod-product-compliance
Lightning Source LLC
Chambersburg PA
CBHW071454140726
47997CB00005B/1725